The Sirtfood Diet

Beginners Guide to Burn Fat and Lose Weight with Healthy Recipes

By

Maria Baker

Introduction

Healthy weight loss has been one of the critical health issues that humans have worried about for many years now. Different methods and techniques have been devised and touted to help resolve this issue over time. Among all of these numerous methods, two have stood out over time; dieting and exercises.

Exercises have been the oldest and conventional answer to healthy weight loss and adequate body fitness. Physicians and other medical practitioners have always reiterated the importance of taking some time to exercise the body. They claimed, with scientific explanations and facts, that regular exercise can help healthily shed unnecessary fat. Whole-body fitness and agility are also some of the benefits that have been attributed to exercise.

However, despite the numerous benefits and the medical and scientific backing that exercising has for ensuring weight loss, people are still on the lookout for other methods of healthy weight loss. Somebody can attribute this to many reasons, some of which may include time constraints, slow results, etc.

Most people have to work for many hours of the day within the week. This leaves them with little or no time to spare to carry out a needed exercise to help them reduce their weight. Hence the need to seek other methods of achieving healthy weight loss and general body fitness since the exercising option is not working for a time.

Another reason why some people are still in search of other ways of achieving healthy weight loss is their impatience for results. Medical practitioners did advise that exercising can be a healthy way of shedding unneeded weight. What they may not tell you is that it takes some time for the weight loss effect to start showing. Depending on the routine and exercising intensity, it may take weeks for the body to lose a reasonable amount of unneeded weight through exercising. This waiting time for the matter shedding effect of exercise to show on the body is considered too long for many people. As a result of this, they are in search of a faster and more efficient method of healthy weight loss.

This leads us to the second most popular way to lose weight in a healthy manner; dieting. Dieting has gained popularity over time as a means of reducing weight. It is considered less stressful and faster than exercising since it does not require too much physical exertion and effort. Dieting, however, is in many variants. While there is dieting in the general sense, there are other variants of dieting with different names and processes.

The general dieting which some school of thoughts has referred to as mindful eating. It is a process whereby people pay detailed attention to the type of food they eat. They are required to research adequately the nutritional content of the food they consume. This way, they can stay away from foods that result in weight gain and eat that which helps them reduce weight.

The other variants of dieting have names and dedicated processes. There are many of them, out of which one stands out as the latest, safest and fastest means of losing weight. This diet is referred to as the Sirtfood diet. This chapter will focus on providing you with information about the Sirtfood diet and its numerous health benefits aside from healthy weight loss.

□

Chapter One: What is Sirtfood Diet?

The way dieting has taken over the nutritional health and body fitness discussions in recent times has been alarming, especially with the issue of healthy weight loss. There seems to be a diet that dominates the weight-loss debate at any point in time. As such, nutritionists and doctors have had a regular job at these different periods, sensitize the public about the inherent benefit and risks associated with the diet.

And just like those times, another diet is up for discussion, and I have decided to educate everyone about it by giving all the facts involved, backed by science and medical knowledge. The diet up for discussion this time is the Sirtfood diet.

Sirtfood diet was introduced by two nutritionists, Aidan Goggins and Glen Matten, working in a gym in the United Kingdom. They introduced it in a book they both authored titled the Sirtfood Diet. The popularity of the diet soared more when the rumor came out that popular artist, Adele, achieved her tremendous weight loss through this diet. There was a bit of truth to the rumor because her trainer is a known fan of the Sirtfood diet. Adele was also pictured on the Sirtfood official website with inscriptions stating "Adele's top secret fat-melting diet." The Sirtfood diet gained more popularity when also rumored celebrities like Pippa Middleton key into it.

Along with the celebrities' backing, another factor that made the Sirtfood diet talk of the town for a very long time is the fact that the diet allows you to drink red wine and snack on things like dark chocolate while on a diet. Eating and drinking these will not affect the effectiveness of the diet. This sounded like a dream come true for people seeking to shed weight without stress. This means that they don't need to give up their favourites because of a weight-shedding diet.

However, associated with this popularity are questions about the safety, benefits, and effectiveness of the diet. These questions and concerns are well-founded as we have witnessed some diet with promises of weight loss turn out to be harmful to various people after the verdicts of medical practitioners. To this end, we will discuss all that you need to know about the Sirtfood diet in this chapter.

The Sirtfood diet is different from all other types of diet as its idea is based on the actions of sirtuins. Sirtuins are classes of proteins that are present in the human body with the function of controlling will discuss all that you need to know about the Sirtfood diet-specific body processes, including metabolism and inflammation. Hence Sirtfood diet involves eating foods that can help trigger this class of protein. When these proteins are activated, they help incite the process of weight loss within the body. Not only do these foods trigger the action of these proteins, but they also aid their production in the body. The presence of these proteins in the body in large quantities is responsible for the speedy rate of weight loss. These food items that help induce the action of these sirtuins are referred to as Sirt foods.

A common of all Sirtfoods is that they are rich in a substance known as polyphenols. These polyphenols are responsible for the production and action of sirtuins. When a considerable amount of polyphenols are present in the body, they react in the body mimicking the effect of prolonged fasting and exercise. These effects then trigger the production of the sirtuin proteins.

We should also note that the diet also involves some forms of reduction in intake. This reduction in calories also speeds up the production of sirtuins. Moreover, removal of the calorie intake reduces the production of glucose and glycogen, which are the body's primary source of energy. Due to the decrease in their production, the body turns to the excess fat in the body as a source of energy. The burning of excess fat in the body as a source of fuel is a means of reducing weight loss. When this process is combined with the production of sirtuin and its effect on the body, a fast rate of weight loss is achieved.

These processes are basically the science behind the Sirtfood diet. Although little research has been carried out on these processes, they are simple biological processes that place in the body. While many have questioned the effectiveness and safety of the Sirtfood Diet, the response seems to be lying in wait in the book written by the proponents of the diet. This response is in the form of a study carried out on about 39 participants at the gym where the authors work. The study stated that these 39 people started the Sirtfood diet. After a week, the average weight loss amongst all participants amounted to a total of 7 pounds, which is approximately 3.2 kg. This result is incredible and almost unbelievable. What makes the results more interesting is the fact that the participants witnessed this weight loss without any form of muscle loss. Some participants were reported to have gained some muscle mass during the weight shedding process.

This result proves that the Sirtfood diet is a better option for some other methods, which the restriction of calories alone. This is because the reduction in calories leads to the burning of body fat and muscle mass for the provision of energy, as explained before. Hence, a Sirtfood diet is able to achieve weight loss without any form of muscle mass loss.

The phases involved in the Sirtfood diet are two. These two phases span for a total of three weeks. This is another striking fact about the Sirtfood diet. Unlike most other diets that take a relatively long time, the Sirtfood diet only lasts for three weeks. During these three weeks, the body is subjected to an intensive Sirtfood diet. After the three weeks, the proponents of the diet advised that it is beneficial to continue eating Sirtfoods so as to sustain the effect of the diet. This is also a plus as the Sirtfoods, apart from being instrumental to the production of sirtuins, are also rich in numerous and varying types of nutrients.

Therefore, continuing their intake with spell good fortune for your health and body fitness.

The phases of the diet include one week of eating Sirtfoods coupled with severe calorie reduction and two weeks of complete Sirtfood meals. The first phase, which is the week of calorie reduction and Sirtfood meals, involves the restriction of the daily calorie intake to 1000 every day for the early three days of the first week.

Also, Sirtfood dieters are to take one Sirtfood meal in conjunction with three green juices every day for the first three days of that week. This menu ends after the early three days of the first week, which ushers in a change in diet. After the first three days, the daily calorie intake is increased to 1500 every day. Also, the Sirtfood meals are now intensified to two Sirtfood meals per day and two green juices. This menu is then maintained until the end of the week, which will signify the start of the second phase of the diet.

The second phase of the diet involves a whole Sirtfood meal with no restriction. The two weeks will feature the three Sirtfood meals per day and one green juice. There is no stated amount of calories to be consumed at this stage. At this point, you will have lost a considerable amount of weight. The second stage is planned to allow you to lose more weight but at a more relaxed rate, hence the lax on the calorie reduction rule. By the end of the two weeks, considerable weight loss will be recorded. This and numerous remarkable health benefits (which will be discussed later) will be noticed in the body.

However, despite this result, the proponents of the diet advised that the diet be continued after the three weeks duration of the diet. While this continuation will not entail complete and strict Sirtfood meals, it is recommended that Sirtfoods are incorporated into the food plan every day. This will help you maintain the beneficial effects of the diet and also nourish the body with vital nutrients obtainable in the Sirtfood items.

There are, however, some downsides to the Sirtfood diet. From the side effects to warnings from health practitioners, there are some things that you should note before starting the Sirtfood diet.

Starting with the side effects, you should note that during the first few days of starting the diet, you may notice some side effects. These side effects are everyday occurrences that succeed in any dietary change in the body. They are usually caused by the reduction of some substances (such as calories) in the body, and these effects are the body's way of reacting to this change. Examples of the side effects include dizziness, nausea, irritability, and incessant hunger.

Another point you may want to worry about is the fact that most medical professionals would not give the diet a thumbs up. While they accept that the diet has a lot of health benefits, the fact that the research and studies on a diet are not much is one reason for their reservations. There are also claims that the calorific reduction and the excess consumption of some of the Sirtfoods may have adverse effects on the body.

Sirtfood items, meals, and recipes are essential topics for discussion. Now that you know what the Sirtfood diet is and how to go about it, there is a need to discuss what food items you need to get and meals that you can make with them.

Sirtfoods are food items that are rich in polyphenol. They range from vegetables to fruits and everyday food items. Famous examples include onions, soy, blueberries, kale, dark chocolate, walnuts, turmeric, and many more. Drinks that are Sirtfood friendly are red wine, coffee, and green tea. You can also add food items such as Bird's eye chili, buckwheat, lovage, and red chicory as part of the Sirtfood items.

Some numerous recipes and delicacies can be made from these food items. These recipes are fascinating and delicious that you may be carried away and forget you are on a diet. This does not, however, affect the nutritional benefits associated with the food. The scope of this book does not allow for the detailed description and guidelines for cooking these Sirtfood – inspired meals. However, there are some popular meals that can try out. They include:

1.   Miso-marinated baked cod and stir-fried greens and sesame
2.   Chicken Breast spiced with kale and onions/tomato and chilli
3.   Tabbouleh (strawberry buckwheat)

Green juice is also an essential part of the Sirtfood diet. The juice basically involves juicing the leafy greens in the Sirtfood group. Kale is usually the favored option, and green apples, lemon juice, or ginger can be added to it for taste.

Health benefits of the Sirtfood diet

There are many benefits that you stand the chance of gaining by starting and adopting the Sirtfood diet. These benefits are essential to a healthy lifestyle and disease-free health. Below are some of the advantages associated with the adoption of the Sirtfood diet.

Healthy weight loss

This is the primary and most crucial advantage that you will enjoy when you adopt the Sirtfood diet. As a matter of fact, it is the primary reason why most people start the Sirtfood diet. And of course, with the reviews and results given by people who have tried the diet in the past, it can be said to new entrants that their hopes will not be dashed.

The Sirtfood diet helps the shedding of weight safely and healthily. This effect, when added to the action of the sirtuins that are triggered into action by the Sirtfoods, the body is then made to burn fat in a way that does not affect the body in a harmful way. The absence of muscle loss further reiterates it during the weight shedding process.

The Sirtfood diet is not only safe but records an impressively fast rate of weight shedding or reduction. According to the study published in the official Sirtfood diet book, the participants in the survey lost as much as seven pounds within seven days of starting the diet. Others who have adopted the diet have also reported a far more impressive result after the completion of the diet.

The Sirtfood diet stands out as a viable means of weight loss based on these two reasons; fast result and safety. Moreover, the fact that it does not require strenuous effort, as in the case of exercising, makes it very appealing. It is thus perfect for people who are busy and cannot afford to exercise frequently. This should not be mistaken to imply that the Sirtfood diet does not support the exercise. Some health professionals recommend that activities be combined with the Sirtfood diet so as to maximize the benefits of the diet. However, the point made in this paragraph is that without exercising, the weight loss benefits of the diet will be still be achieved.

Another upside to the weight loss benefit of the diet is the fact that it does not involve extremities and strict food restrictions, as seen in other types of diet. You are still at liberty to enjoy your dark chocolates and drink red wines at parties and occasions while on the Sirtfood diet. You can even take your cup of coffee every morning before going to work while enjoying the benefits of the Sirtfood diet. Moreover, there are many delicious and savoury recipes that can be made from the Sirtfood items. These recipes are so inviting and nutritious that you won't have a feeling that you are on a diet. All of these 'indulgences' are not available with most diets as they prescribe strict dietary requirements.

Reduction of the risk of diabetes

Diabetes is a dangerous ailment that affects the human body as a result of excess sugar in the blood and, by extension, the inadequacy of insulin to control and convert the sugar to glucose.

One of the significant aspects of the Sirtfood diet is the reduction of daily calorie intake for several days. While this is not enough to sustainably reduce the level of blood sugar in the body, the aftermath of the reduction is what matters. By reducing the calorie intake for a while, the rate of metabolism in the body, which is a significant determinant of the number of calories needed, reduces. Due to this, the number of calories required by the body is substantially reduced. Hence the sugar ingested is thus reduced, lowering the risk of diabetes.

The disclaimer that needs to accompany this point is that this effect will remain valid as long as there is no increase in the number of calories taken by the person. If this happens (i.e., the calorie intake increases), it can result in some health issues.

Provision of needed nutrients for the body

The body is provided with large quantities of many important nutrients during the Sirtfood diet. This is because the Sirtfoods, apart from being rich in polyphenol and sirtuins activators, are also highly nutritious foods that are loaded with immense amounts of nutrients. Eating these foods even after the completion of the diet, will do the body a whole lot of good. The Sirtfood group includes different classes of food items such as vegetables and fruits. These are known to contain a considerable amount of mineral salts necessary for the production of enzymes and hormones. These enzymes and hormones are required for the optimal functioning of the body. Therefore, apart from loading the body with nutrients, the Sirtfood diet also ensures the optimal performance of the body system.

Energy-Boosting effect

Some studies have indicated that the Sirtfood diet also increases the energy of the body. This effect is, however, linked to the action of the numerous nutrients present in the Sirtfood items.

Lowers the risk of heart issues and inflammation

The sirtuins, which are the vital substance in the Sirtfood diet, have also been proven to reduce the risk of inflammation in mammals. Adopting and sticking to the Sirtfood diet will further increase the production of sirtuins and, by extension, lowers the risk of inflammation.

Some Sirtfood such as dark chocolate has been studied and touted to reduce the risk of heart diseases.

□

Chapter Two: Top Sirtfoods

Sirtuins are great in regulating our metabolic system, which makes it feasible to control and stay healthy while burning fat. One primary function of sirtuins is to help revive energy sensors in our cells, providing a replicate when they are shortages during fasting and exercising. While these activities trigger the sirtuin's genes, these most times come with much pressure and responsibilities hard to keep. The following are top Sirtfoods which present an impressive list of superfoods that foster a healthy living style. After eating one or more of these top Sirt foods, you will realize that having a healthier body is possible without going through some rigorous fast and exercise.

1) The Buck Wheat: The buckwheat is the most preferred Sirt foods. As the name implies, the buckwheat is not related to the Wheat in any way. The buckwheat is a grain that belongs to the surreal and rhubarb plants' family. Buckwheats are mostly used in making teas like the Buck Wheat tea and also in processing items into consumables such as the grouts, flours, and noddles. The grouts from this buckwheat are known to be the primary ingredients for many traditional and European meals. Buckwheats are of two categories, and this includes the common buckwheat and the tertiary buckwheat. The two are quite useful and beneficial both as food and medicines to the body.

Nutritional Value:
- Calories: 340-343.
- Protein: 9-10%.
- Carbs: 13-2g.
- Sugar: 0g.
- Fibre: 10g.
- Fat: 3.40g.266.

Health Benefits:
1. It helps improve heart health.
2. It cut down calories, thereby reducing blood sugar.
3. It's non-allergic and gluten-free, perfect for folks with Celia disaster.

4.   Highly rich in dietary fibre for easy digestion of food.

5.   It helps fight against cancers.

2) Birds Eye Chilies: The bird-eye chili pepper, also known as the olives, is used regularly by the southeast Asian and Europeans when making cuisine. The bird-eye chilli often grows in hot weather conditions. These sauce chilies are often known by its ability to make potent heat, which is used as spices when making dishes or fiery sauces; apart from spicing things up, it is remarkably known for its weight reduction abilities.

Nutritional values:

- No. of calories 18.
- No. of fat 0-2g.
- No. of cholesterol 0.mg.
- No. of sodium 4mg.
- No. of potassium 45mg.
- No. of carbohydrates 4g.
- Total carbohydrates 4gram.
- No of dietary fibre 0.7gram.
- No of protein 0.8gram
- Vitamin A: present 2%.
- Calcium presents 0%.
- Vitamin E: 2%.
- Niacin: 4%.
- Magnesium: 20%.
- Vitamin C: 72%.
- Ion 0%.
- Zinc.

Health benefits:

1.   It helps in easy digestion.

2.   It helps fasten the healing process of stomach ulcers.

3.   It can act as a remedy for arthritis and rheumatism.

4.   It helps reduced blood cholesterol and blood pressure.

3) Capers: Capers is known for its spicy and unique taste to Italian dishes. There are mostly used as seasonings for spicy dishes. Aside from its flourishing and tangy taste, they also have lots of nutrients that are beneficial to our health.

Nutritional Value for 100 grams:

- Carbs 5g.

- Sugar 0.4g.
- Fiber 3g.
- Fat 0.9g.
- Protein 2g.
- Vitamin C, 4g.
- Vitamin A138g.
- Vitamin K, 246mg.
- Vitamin E 0.88mg.
- Niacin 0.6 5mg.
- Riboflavin 0.1mg.
- Sodium 2960mg.
- Potassium 40mg.
- Energy contains 961g.

Health Benefits:

1.   It protects against free radicals, which causes cancer of the skin and others.

2.   It helps in strengthening the human bones and teeth.

3.   It contains vitamin A, which increases the eye functionalities to perform better.

4.   It clears and reduces by-products in foods and meat that are prone to cause cancers.

5.   It helps keep the skin moisture.

4) Celery: Celery belongs to the Apiaceae family. This family is a significant constituent for carrots and parsley alongside celeriac. They are also known for their much deposit of water and low calorie, which makes it beneficial to the health.

Nutritional Value:

- 40g of calorie stalk.
- 0.6g of fibre.
- 0.1gram of fat.
- 32mg of sodium.
- 1.2g of carbs.
- 0.5g of sugar.
- 0.3g of protein.

Health Benefits:

1.   It helps prevent oxidation injuries to blood vessels, cells, etc.

2.   Arthritis, osteoporosis are a result of severe inflammation, which the nutrients contain; celery helps reduce it.

3.   It helps reduce the acidic nature or contents in foods.

5) Coffee: Coffee is tagged with its potential ability to boost energy. Aside from that, cocoa contains certain nutrients that are beneficial to us.

Nutritional Value for 100 grams of coffee:

*   Sodium
*   Potassium 92mg.
*   Magnesium 8mg.
*   0.0mg of manganese.
*   0.0mg of riboflavin.
*   0.7 mg of niacin.

Health Benefits:

1.   It protects against diabetes and liver cancer.
2.   It promotes heart health.
3.   It helps regulate fluid balance.

6) Cocoa: The Cocoa, which is mainly used as chocolate, is imbibed with lots of nutrients with a tremendous impact on human health.

Nutritional Value of 100 grams of Cocoa chocolate:

*   The fibre contains 11g.
*   Iron 67%.
*   Magnesium includes 58% (RDI).
*   Copper contains 89% (RDI).
*   Manganese comprises 98% (RDI).
*   With other minerals such as selenium, zinc phosphorous, potassium.

Health Benefits:

1.   It helps reduce blood pressure.
2.   It Combats and lowers every risk of a heart attack.
3.   It enhances brain functions due to active polyphenols.
4.   It helps balance or reduces fats in diverse ways.

7) Extra Virgin Oil: The extra virgin oil is reportedly known as one of the best and healthiest oils across the globe. People who often take this oil have proven experience in good health and healthier lives. The extra olive oil is originated and extracted from the olive fruit. It is one that is done without any chemical or heat.

Nutritional Value for 15g of Virgin Oil (1tbs):

- 14gram of fat.
- 0.3mg of sodium.
- 0g of carbohydrates.
- 0g of Fiber.
- 0g of protein and sugar.

Health Benefits:

1. It supports and enhances nerve conduction.
2. It is rich in vitamin K, which makes it perfect for blood clotting.
3. It helps protect heart health.

8) Green Tea Virgin: Green tea is known for its distinctive weight loss abilities. Green tea is among the most famous tea worldwide. It comes in different varieties such as matcha green tea and other brewed green tea.

Nutritional Value:

- 306mg of protein.
- 272mg of amino acid.
- 50mg of lipid.
- Potassium 27mg.
- Magnesium (2.3mg).
- Calcium 4.2mg.
- Zinc 0.62mg.
- Phosphorous 3.5mg.
- 0.17mg of iron.
- It also contains vitamins A, B1, B2, B6, C, E, and K.

Health Benefits:

1. It promotes weight loss.
2. It protects the cells from damage
3. It regulates blood sugar levels
4. It enhances focus and relaxation

9) Kale: kales are green vegetables that are associated with the mustard family. There are rich in nutrients and other minerals.

Nutritional Value:

- For 100gram
- DV: Daily value
- 49, calories
- 0.9g of fat (DV)
- 0mg of cholesterol
- 38mg of sodium
- 4.0gram of protein
- One-ninety-nine percent of vitamin A (DV)
- Fifteen per cent of Calcium (DV)
- Zero per cent of Vitamin D (DV)
- Zero per cent of Cobalamin (DV)
- Two-hundred per cent of Vitamin C (DV)
- Eight per cent of Iron (DV)
- Fifteen per cent of vitamin B-6 (DV)

Health Benefits:

1. It helps develop and enhance the brain due to its high intake of folate and vitamins
2. Nutrients such as the lutein or Zeaxanthins helps fight against cataracts in human health
3. It helps regulate our blood sugar.

10) Lovage: The Lovage plant is a plant that belongs to the dill and carrots family. The Lovage plants are usually green in colour depicting the cilantro and parsley shape. The Lovage leave has a powerful scent, which makes its roots leaves more useful for medical purpose.

Nutritional Value:

- 5g of carbs
- 3g of fibre
- 4g of sugar
- 0g of fat
- 3gram of protein
- 80mg of sodium
- 400mg of potassium
- 0mg of cholesterol

- Eighty –three per cent of Vitamin A (daily intake)
- Forty-three per cent of calcium (daily intake)
- Fifteen per cent of calcium (daily intake)
- Fifteen per cent of Iron (daily intake)

Health Benefits:

1. It helps fight against harmful organisms in the body.
2. It protects against the effects of an allergy.
3. It helps the digestive process, thereby alleviating and neutralizing stomach upset.
4. Lovage contains a too high compound that can very quickly desiccate rough spots or wounds in our body. These compounds include limonene, quercetin, and Eugene.
5. Its properties can also be beneficial to the care of our skin. When the lovage leaves are correctly applied to the skin, it helps reduce every skin related problem such as acne, psoriasis, wrinkles, and quite a number of them, making smooth the surface of our skin.

11) Medjool Dates: Medjool dates contain a lot of sugar in its food. It also consists of other minerals like fibres and vitamins. The Medjool dates are dried fruits that richly contain calories for each date.

Nutritional Value for 48 grams of Medjool Dates:

- 2% of calcium (Du).
- 133 calories
- 36g of carbs
- 3.2g of Fiber
- 0.8g protein
- 32g of sugar
- 2% of iron (Daily intake)
- 7% of potassium
- 19% of copper
- Vitamin B6, 7%
- Magnesium, 6%

Health Benefits:

1. It helps regulate blood sugar levels.
2. The presence of magnesium (180gram) helps reduce blood sugar levels.
3. The presence of chlorine (2mg) helps boost the brain functions in man.

4.	It helps strengthens the body due to the high number of carbs.

12) Parsley: The Parsley comes with lots of health benefits that help both dieters and non-dieters sustain their health.

Nutritional Value:

- For two tablespoons
- Two calories
- 12% of vitamin A (daily intake)
- 16% of vitamin C
- 154% of vitamin K

Health benefits:

1.	Parsley reduces the risk of breast and skin cancers.
2.	It combats against disease.
3.	It keeps the blood vessels immune from others.
4.	It fights against inflammation.

13) Red Chicory: The red chicory, also called the Italian chicory or chicorium it's often mistaken for red cabbage by most dieters. It has a distinctive taste, which makes it ideal for all Italian dishes. The red chicory is purely different from other vegetables, and it is rich in vitamin K, copper, and zinc, yet low in calories.

Nutritional Value:

- 2-cup of red chicory
- 20 calorie
- 0g of fat
- 4g of carbs
- 1g of fibre
- Three per cent of iron (Daily intake)
- Five per cent of zinc (Daily intake)
- Thirty per cent of copper(Daily intake)
- Five per cent of phosphorous
- Five per cent of potassium
- One seventy per cent of Vitamin K
- Seven per cent of Vitamin C
- Three per cent of vitamin B6

Health Benefits:

1.	It enhances our bone structures.
2.	It regulates the blood sugars in our body with the help of inulin fibre.

3.   It helps ease and improve our digestive system.

14) Red Onion: Onions are among the most vital vegetables for growth and weight loss. They contain vitamins, minerals, and plants compound, which helps in building the human body. Onions are used to treat headaches, mouth sores, and other trivial ailments in times past. Onions are not only beneficial as food ingredients but also useful in Sirtfoods diets because of their nutrients.

Nutritional Value:

Servings: 1 for 100 grams.

- 85 calories
- 4, sodium
- 127 of manganese.
- Carb, 2.6g.
- Vitamin A, D, and calcium

Health Benefits:

1.   It helps boost heart health.

2.   It helps prevent high blood pressure.

3.   It contains anthocyanins, which helps prevents diabetes tumours, and cancers.

4.   Onions also help strengthen the body system and gut.

15) Red wine: The red wine constitutes resveratrol, which is an ideal drink to take in place of high alcohol drinks.

Nutritional Value:

Servings: 1 for 100 grams.

- 40%of floricide
- 100% of manganese
- 5% of potassium
- 4% of vitamin B6
- 3% of vitamin B2
- 2% of chlorine

Health Benefits:

1.   It helps boost energy in the body.

2.   Enhance the flow of oxygen in the body.

3.   It improves brain functionalities.

4.   It helps reduce tooth decay.

16) Rocket: Rocket, which is also known as arugula, consists of various vital nutrients, some of which include high nitrates leaves, vitamin C, vitamin K, and A.

Health Benefits:
1.   It helps fight against cancer.
2.   It increases eyesight levels.
It contains vitamin K, which enhances the heart, bones, and skin health.
17) Soy: The soy, also known as the soya beans, comes from beans. The powder, soy milk, and soy protein all came from the soy.
Nutritional Value for 100 grams of soya Bean:
*   173 calories
*   62% of water
*   16.5g of protein
*   9.89g of carbohydrates
*   3g of sugar
*   6g of Fiber
Health Benefits:
1.   It helps in the prevention of cancer, in most cases, breast cancer. People who consumed soy have less risk of having breast cancer.
2.   It helps prevent diabetes. Soy contains fiber and protein, which drastically reduces our blood sugar levels.
3.   It helps reduced diarrhoea. A mixture of soy fiber with rehydration solution goes a long way in relieving diarrhoea.
4.   It combats high blood pressure. By just eating soy protein, high blood pressure can be reduced.
5.   It helps reduce breast pain. Regular drinking of soy milk has been confirmed in the reduction of breast pain.
18) Strawberries: Strawberries are among the top Sirtfoods with powerful antioxidants content. There are sweet, refreshing, and nourishing. The strawberry contains low calories, which makes it perfect and suitable for people with diabetes or those who prefer to mix with any diet. It contains vitamin C, potassium, and folic acid. These nutrients are what builds and support the functioning of the human body.
Nutritional Value:
*   53 calories.
*   1.1g of protein
*   12.7g of carbs
*   3.30g of Fiber

- 27mg of calcium
- 0.68mg of iron
- 22mg of magnesium
- 40mg of phosphorous
- 254 potassium
- 97.6mg of vitamin
- 40mg of folic

Health Benefits:

1. It reduces every form of heart disease to occur.
2. It helps fight against strokes.
3. It curbs every effect of cancers due to its powerful antioxidants.
4. It has the potency to reduce high blood pressure due to its healthy potassium contents.

19) Turmeric: The turmeric, also known as the golden spice, is a huge plant that is grown in Asia countries. Turmeric is a spice used categorically for meals in diverse ways.

Nutritional Value for 1-tbsp:

- Calories 29
- Protein 0.3g
- Fat 0.3g
- Carbs 6.3gram
- Fibre 2.0gram
- Sugar 0.31gram
- Manganese 26%
- Potassium 5%
- Vitamin C: 3%

Health Benefits:

1). It helps relieve all kinds of pain, including arthritis.
2). It increases the life expectancy rate of the liver due to its antioxidants abilities.
3). It fights against cancer.
4). It aids the easy digestion of food in humans.

20) Walnuts: Walnuts are Sirtfoods usually eaten on their own as snacks. They are known to be low on sodium, sugar with excessive nutrients. The Walnut, when taken, helps cut down the effects of blood pressure in our body, thereby improving the human heart and brain health.

Nutritional Value:
- It contains 65% fat and 15%protein
- High in fibre, low in carbs.
- You get the following nutritional value for one ounce of nuts (30gram).
- 185: calories
- 40% of water
- 4.3g of protein 3.9g of carbohydrates
- 0.7g of sugar.18.5g of fat
- 1.9g of fibre
- Vitamins Include; Copper, folic acid, phosphorous, vitamin B6, magnesium.

Health Benefits:

1). Studies have proved that eating nuts can improve heart health.

2). It helps combats rare diseases leading to cancer.

3). It helps boost our brain functions.

4). It fights against depression and ageing in humans.

Chapter Three: Sirtfood diet to burn fat and lose weight

The various process involves in burning fat in Sirtfoods includes; the soup diet, the Dukan Diet, and 5.2 diets. This diet method has yielded the possible results in the lives of many who are in dire need to burn fat. Among others is the famous celebrity known as Adele, who used the Sirt diet food to burn 7lbs of fat within a short time-space. Here is what you need to know about burning fat and what foods to use.

Cabbage Soup Diet

The cabbage soup diet is one effective method to help lose weight fast. Irrespective of your awful experience in using other ways to lose weight with no possible results, this cabbage soup diet has little or no doubt on why you shouldn't lose weight.

Unlike the less famous diet plan, the cabbage soup diet has been around for years, used by dieters around the world, and has been testified to make people lose 10 pounds in a concise space. Now that you know how effective the cabbage soup diet is, it's time to go through the process of using this Sirtfood and the various health risk and factors to consider for significant results.

Cabbage Soup Diet: What it is

The diet method is a simple process that allows you to spend an average of 7 days taking in an immeasurable amount of low-calorie cabbage soup, fully cooked and prepared by you. Which makes the cabbage soup becomes your diet for that period. During this period, you're allowed to eat other foods like fruit and the rest, but the amount of food to eat must be in small quantities in order not to alter the process of losing fat in a quicker time frame. Individuals who take up this diet plan has claimed to burn fat as much as 10lbs in the space of 7 days. How does it work?

The cabbage soup diet plan has little fat with an incredibly high fibre diet. This, in turn, offers you a zero calories cabbage soup in which eating too much of it only makes you lose weight.

The Diet recipe

Five Large onions (sliced)

Two peppers (green) Chopped

Two cans of tomatoes

Sliced Mushroom (preferably, 250g)

One bunch of celery, slashed

Half cabbage,

sliced

 A dry onion mixed with soup

Two cubes of bouillon, Inclusive; salt & pepper.

Additional ingredients when adding flour include;

Cayenne pepper

Curry powder

Mixed herbs and other unique seasonings.

Instructions:

Sauté the sliced onions with spray oil in a cooking pot.

Add the chopped green peppers and warm for two minutes.

The celery, mushroom, cabbage leaves, and carrots should be added after heating.

Add a pinch of cayenne pepper.

Twelve cups of water plus any other stock cubes will be added.

Cook food on moderate heat till vegetables are soft and the soup is of suitable viscosity.

The perfect meal plan for cabbage soup diet

Day 1: Indefinite consumption of cabbage soup alongside fruits and water. Bananas and sugar-filled juice should be avoided.

Day 2: Cabbage soup plus vegetables. Dinner meal; potatoes plus butter excluding fruits.

Day 3: Cabbage soup alongside fruits or vegetables of your choice. Avoid potatoes and bananas.

Day 4: Consume a large amount of cabbage soup with milk and bananas (up to 7).

Day5:

An immeasurable amount of cabbage soup, beef plus tomatoes. Don't forget to drink 8-9 glasses of water to cleanse your system from uric acid.

Day6: Consume as much cabbage soup as you can plus beef and vegetables.

Day7: Consume as much cabbage soup you can with a small portion of brown rice, fruit juice, and vegetables. Note: Fruit juice must be sugar-free.

Benefits of the Cabbage Soup Diet

The cabbage soup diet plan is perfect for most peeps because it's ridiculously cheap and poise to be a great diet meal to take for a quicker result. These Sirtfoods can be used when making out for special events such as the wedding, grand ceremonial, or confidential event. Looking at its short timeframe (7days), when duly followed, has the potency to yield remarkable results. Aside from that, cabbage has its nutritional benefits. It contains a high amount of fiber, antioxidants, and vitamin C, which makes it beneficial to our health.

Drawbacks of the Cabbage soup diet.

We've heard critics said the weight loss plan is a mirage because they believed you're losing water rather than losing fat, which makes you more susceptible to gain excess weight when you begin your usual diet. The case of achieving your weight back after going through the cabbage food diet is real for some persons, majorly a few people, because the diet tends to be low in calories with zero protein resulting in less body fat to more water and muscle loss. We know you don't want that to happen because this book aims to lose body fat/weight and permanently and not gain them back. While following the cabbage soup diet plan, the best way to maintain your weight loss and not gain them is to supplement the soup with a small portion of protein. Adding proteins like the rye bread and other unique flavors will annul every effect of quickly regaining your fat when you begin the standard diet.

In case you're not comfortable with the cabbage soup diet plan, the 5:2 diet or Dukan diet plan will most probably be your best fit.

The 5:2 Diet plan

5:2 diet plans are the most straightforward diet plan to undertake. The process includes reducing your calorie intake to 500 for two straight days a week while eating your usual diet plan the remaining days a week. When on the 5:2 diet plan, we recommend not to eat takeaways but rather to keep your daily calorie intake. The recommended calorie intakes are 2000 for women and 2500 for men.

How it works

The 5:2 diet plan is just another name for regular intermittent fasting. This is a more effective way of losing weight because it's a process that limits your calorie intake gradually than doing it all at once. This method shifts your body system to function in the repair mode rather than the stiff starvation mode.

The recipes

The following recipes will help you stay in check, not exceeding the 500 calories daily intake.

Meal Plan for 5:2 diet.

- Banana oat muffins
- Serves: 12
- No. of Calories for each muffin 219
- Prep. Time: 17 minutes
- Cooking time: About 30 minutes
- 350calories of 100g oats
- 155calories of whole-wheat flour (50g)
- 503 calories of white flour (150g)
- Ten calories of two tablespoons of baking powder
- Five calories of 1 tablespoon bicarbonate of soda.
- Salt ¼
- Three hundred calories of sugar, 75gram of Muscovado.
- Four hundred eighty calories of mashed, four pieces of bananas.
- One egg
- 5 tbsp. Olive oil (light) 500 calories.
- 173-185calories of sunflower seeds mix with pumpkin

Cooking instructions

1. Preheat oven continuously until it's averagely heated. Preferably 180 degrees.
2. Place a 12-hole muffin tin alongside its paper cases.

3.   The oats, flours, baking powder, salt, sugar, and bicarbonate should be thoroughly mixed.

4.   The following, such as egg, oil, and mashed bananas, will be fiercely mixed and poured into the dry oat and flour.

5.   Add a spoon to the ready-made muffin and stir the top of each muffin with its seed and oats.

6.   It is cooked until it's brown and springy at sight. Baking time/cooking time should be 20-minutes long.

Cod Provencal Meal.

Servings: 2

247 Calories for each serves.

Prep. Time: 10min

Cooking time: 23minutes

Ingredients:

- One red pepper, sliced 30 calorie
- One yellow pepper, sliced (30cal)
- 34 cal. Of one courgette, it is chopped.
- Pepper and salt
- One cal. of cooking spray
- (2*150g) of Cod fillets, it must be peeled. 280 calorie.
- Cherry tomato (100gram), calorie: 18
- Black Olives, thoroughly rinsed. 30gram, 9 cal.
- 9 cal. Of half lemon with juice
- Thyme leaves, 5 cal.

Cooking Guide

1) Heat the oven at an average of 200c/400f/ Gmask mark6.

2) Put the sliced pepper, onions, and courgettes in a dish.

3) Sprinkle one calorie of cooking spray alongside seasoned salt and pepper.

4) Fry/roast for about 8-1 minutes.

5) Ensure to put the cod fillet on top.

6) Sprinkle one calorie of cooking spray alongside tomatoes, lemon zest, and olives at the surface of fish and stir a little.

7) Squeeze the lemon juice while spraying with herbs season.

8) Cooked till it becomes dense(white colour). This takes about 10-12 minutes of cooking time.

9) Serve food immediately after stirring with olives.

The Mexican Bean Burgers

Servings: 4 - calories for each serving: 245

Prep Time: 15-20 minutes.
Cooking Time: 23 minutes
Ingredients:
*   One calorie of cooking spray.
*   Half red onion, skinned, removed, and sliced.19calorie.
*   Four spring onions perfectly chopped. Six calories.
*   Two garlic (cloves), chopped. Eight calories.
*   One big size chilli (red), perfectly sliced 8-10calorie.desseded.
*   Two tablespoons of Mexican 8 calorie.
*   One and a half ×400g can of beans, mixed. 350 calories.
*   One piece of egg, 79 calories.
*   Bread crumbs (50g) 130 calories.
*   Two tablespoons of coriander leaves (sliced) 10calories.
*   Half lime of fruit juice five calories.
*   75gram of feta cheese (low fat) 134 calories.
*   80gram of halloumi cheese, 200 calories.
*   Sliced pepper.
*   Salt.

Cooking Guide

1. Place a frying pan on the oven with one calorie of cooking spray.
2. Spices such as the spring onions, sliced pepper, salt should be added to the frying pan over an average of heat for six minutes till it gets soft and not coloured.
3. Allow cooling for about three minutes before adding bread crumbs, lime juice, and egg. Allow to seasoned before mixing.
4. Stir softly in the crumbled feta.
5. Wash hands in water, allow drying for two minutes before shaping the mixture into your desired patties (four preferably).
6. Cool in the fridge for 15-20minutes to firm up.
7. Again preheat the grill to moderate heat for about 3minutes. Then spray a little amount of cooking oil in frying pan and cook till it turns golden brown.
8. Remove and serve the meal.

Benefits of this diet plan

The 5:2 diet plan is one of the most uncomplicated Sirtfood plans to undergo; aside from its simplicity, it also comes with benefits that help boost cognitive functions, fighting against severe health conditions like Alzheimer's and dementia. This diet plan seems easy to most dieters because it's the only plan that allows you fast one day at a time just to maintain weight loss.

The diet plan also helps adjust our eating plan if the 5:2 diet plan has been carrying on for a long time. We may tend to adapt to the 5:2 diet plan, thereby adjusting our eating habits. Different people have often time discussed their experience with the 5:2 diet plan, some of which the backgrounds are of tremendous help to dieters. The project has made some individuals halt every quick urge for food and consuming or limiting their calorie consumption levels.

The 5:2 diet plans also help you save more money while still consuming your favourite delicate.

Tips to note:

The following tips will help you embark on this 5:2 diet plan virtually without breaking its rules.

High-quality flavours with low calories:

During this period, it's advisable not to mix carbs. Lower your calorie level because high-calorie intake will stir hunger in you, making you famished by 10 am. When going through this process, put your focus more on eating salads, tofu, fish, sugar-free juice, or vegetables. Also, you can step it up with herbs, flavours, and other spices. By adding some chilli cakes in soups or baked stew will go a long way in spicing your dishes.

Know your perfect mealtime

People who eat breakfast early usually feel less hungry for the day. Unfortunately, people doing the 5:2 diet plans realize that the later we eat, the less hungry we become. It's up to you to determine the best mealtime that is most suitable for you.

Dukan Diet

The Dukan diet is a plan tailored specifically for weight loss and how to maintain that loss for a long time or a lifetime. The program is modelled in such a way that you're allowed to eat certain kinds of food that are low in carbohydrate and high in protein. The Dukan diet plan is categorized into four phases, and these phases include the "attack and cruise" phase as well as the "consolidation and stabilization phase." The goal of the first-two phase is on weight loss, while the last-two steps aim at sustaining that loss.

Attack Phase: This phase focuses on cutting down on all non-protein meals fostering its capacity to lose fat in a quicker timeframe. During this period, you focus more on eating pure protein. Pure proteins to consider during this phase include fish, lean meat, eggs, and tofu. As there is no limitation to what you can eat, eating only pure protein might sound weird but be rest assured you can never go hungry because the results accrued to this process are nothing compared to the process. The attack phase usually takes two-three days to accomplish.

Cruise Phase: The cruise phase: This phase presents the use of approved vegetables freshly. For this phase, you have the choice to select all proteins and vegetables with a mix as your preferred meal. It is something you keep doing till your aim is fully accomplished, which takes four to five days to lose a pound.

The consolidation phase: The consolidation, which is the third phase, slowly presents new foods into the body system, which helps adjust the body into a more desirable lifestyle. The meals introduced to our system include fresh fruits, cheese, dessert, and wholegrain.

The stabilization stage: The stabilization is the fourth stage of the Dukan plan. At this stage, our body is gradually returning to its usual balanced diet because the process of losing weight has already been accomplished. This stage helps enlightened us on the lessons learned, the dos and don'ts of weight loss, and how to self-regulate on our usual diet plan. At this stage, there are only three simple rules to follow, and this includes; eating one-protein a day every week, using the staircase and not the lift, and taking 3-4 tablespoon of oat bran each day. As easy as they sound, some dieters still fail to observe the rules or processes of each stage. Should in case you forget or cheat at any stage, just take on a few more natural pure protein days to retrace your steps back on the diet plan. No matter what the goal is, the Dukan diet plan will simplify the weight loss process, making you attain your right weight with ease.

Dukan Diet Recipes

The Piri Piri spicy chicken dish

Servings: 4

Ingredients:

- Large chicken thighs eight pieces
- Chilli flakes, two teaspoons
- Two garlic (cloves), sliced.
- Oregano, One teaspoon
- Paprika, One teaspoon Cider Vinegar, One-quarter cup
- Lemon Juice, Half
- Lime juice, half
- Black pepper
- Sea salt

Cooking guide

1. Mix and slightly stir the chili flakes, lemon juice, paprika, vinegar, garlic, and oregano in an average size bowl to get a perfect marinade.

2. Add chicken to the bowl and coat each piece in the marinade.

3. Cover bowl firmly and place in the refrigerator for an extended period, preferably 5 hours or more or over the night.

4. Remove bowl from the fridge and pull out the chicken from the marinade.

5.   Ensure the chicken is seasoned averagely with salt and pepper to taste.
6.   Cook thoroughly on moderate heat.
7.   If you're on the Dukan diet plan, we recommend you peeled off the skin.
8.   Serve your Piri Piri spicy chicken dish with lime juice or plain fat-free yoghurt.
There is no particular kind of food for this diet; what matters is the number of calories present in each meal. That is, any food or feed to be taken must not exceed its limit.

Chapter Four: How it works and how it is structured

The Sirt diet plan has two corresponding processes that span three weeks to get done. After this, you're free to continue eating as many Sirt food alongside your meal. There are specific recipes to include during this stage, but you can get these recipes in the recipes section of the book. The meals included are mainly Sirtfoods and other recipes. The major ingredients included for the Sirtfood weight loss process include the matcha green tea powder, buckwheat, and Lova. The Sirtfoods, green juice is a whole game-changer when it comes to the structuring of your diet plan. The green juice is one you will have to prepare at least one to four times daily to yield its effect. Preparing the green juice requires you to get a juicer and a kitchen scale. It's advised not to use a blender because using one won't be effective.

The Green Juice

Kale, 75g.

Arugula, 30g. (1oz)

Parsley, 5g.

Celery, two sticks.

Ginger, 1gm

A green apple, half

Lemon, half

Matcha green tea, A half teaspoon

When these ingredients are ready, juice them together, excluding the green tea powder with lemon, and pour them into a large cup. Squeeze the juice from the lemon and pour alongside the green tea powder into the juice. Remember, the first phase of the green juice serves you for seven days while taking fewer calories and more green juice. This process helps you burn fat to a desirable level, thereby losing seven pounds of weight in a period of seven to eight days. For three non-consecutive days at phase one, you will drink three-juice a day alongside your meal. Note: Calorie intake should not exceed 1000. For each day, you have the choice to select what meal to eat among the varieties included in the Sirtfood plan. Sirtfoods choices to select include tofu, buckwheat, and noodle. Day 4-7, you will take two green juices alongside Sirt food meals per day. The second phase is a phase where you gradually begin to lose weight. In this stage, you still have to take one green juice each day alongside the Sirtfood. This method of weight loss can be repeated again and again until you have reached your desired weight. The green juice process should not be halt, it's advised you continue this process even after you have completed the Sirtfood diet juice process.

Sirtfood Diet Plan - Side Effect

Each phase of the Sirt food diet comes with a lot of benefits and which constitutes of low nutrients and calories. Also, for people with diabetes, they may be some slight changes in their blood sugar level due to the continuous drink of green juice at the beginning of the plan. People without any health challenge may also experience hunger due to the restrictions of calorie intake and the heavy consumption of juice.

Other effects such as fatigue, sightedness may be experienced when you begin the phase one process, but all these won't incur any damage/risk to your health. When you get to the second phase, the effects will be reduced. Besides, only a few people do experience the side effects of the green juice Sirt method.

Chapter Five: Recipes

1.   LAMB BUTTERNUT SQUASH AND DATE TAGINE
Ingredients
*   800g of lamb neck filet (cut into small chunks)
*   400g of tin chopped tomatoes
*   500g of butternut squash
*   400g of drained tin chickpeas
*   100b of pitted and chopped dates
*   Two tablespoons of Olive oil
*   One sliced red onion
*   Grated 2 cm ginger
*   Three Crushed or grated garlic cloves
*   One teaspoon of chili flakes
*   Two teaspoons of cumin seeds
*   One cinnamon stick
*   Two teaspoons of grounded turmeric
*   Half teaspoon of salt
*   Two tablespoons of fresh coriander
Procedures
1.   Preheat the oven to 160 °C.
2.   Sprinkle two tablespoons of olive oil into a large ovenproof saucepan or casserole dish.
3.   Add sliced onion, cover, and allow it to cook on a gentle heat for 5 minutes. Cook the onion until it's softened, not brown.
4.   Next, you add your garlic, chili, cumin, cinnamon, turmeric, and ginger.
5.   Stir the mixture well and leave it open to cook for one minute. You can splash in little water if it's too dry.
6.   Add your lamb chunks and stir well till the meat is well coated with onion and spices. Then, add salt, dates, tomatoes, and about 200ml of water.

7. Pour the tagine into a bowl, cover it, and put in the preheated oven for 1 hour 15 minutes.

8. When it's 30 minutes to the cooking time, add butternut squash and drained chickpea. Then stir it all together and return to the oven to cook for the remaining 30 minutes.

9. Sprinkle coriander for garnish.

10. Serve.

Nutritional information

Servings: 6

Per serving:

Fats 14g

Carbohydrates 40g

Protein 33g

Calories 401kcal

2. PRAWN ARRABBIATA

Ingredients

- 350g of peeled prawns
- 400g of chopped tomatoes
- 400g of dried penne (pasta)
- 400g of tined plum pureed tomatoes
- Two tablespoons of olive oil or low cholesterol oil
- One peeled and finely diced onion
- Three minced garlic cloves
- One teaspoon of salt
- Two tablespoons of tomato paste
- One teaspoon of garlic granules
- Two teaspoons of dried chili flakes, extra for garnish
- 4 cups of water
- A handful of roughly torn Basil leaves
- Shaved or grated Pecorino to serve

Procedures

1. Add half a tablespoon of salt to a large pot of boiling water and cook your penne according to instructions on the pack.

2. Heat your olive oil in a separate pan. Add onion and stir gently over medium-low heat for 4 minutes. It should not turn brown.

3.   Add your minced garlic cloves and let it cook for a few minutes more.
4.   Next, add your pureed tomatoes, tomato paste, and chopped tomatoes and stir.
5.   Then, add your salt, garlic powder, and chili flakes. Use a wooden spoon to crush the chopped tomatoes in the sauce gently.
6.   Allow it to simmer for about 8 minutes while stirring continuously.
7.   Add prawns, stir and cook until the prawns turn pink.
8.   Drain your pasta, pour into the sauce, and stir properly. Then, add your basil leaves.
9.   Garnish with extra chili flakes.
10.   Ready to serve. You can serve yummy prawn arrabbiata with grated or shaved Pecorino.

Nutritional information
Servings: 4
Per serving:
Fats 7g
Carbohydrates 89g
Protein 15g
Calories 487kcal

3.   TUMERIC BAKED SALMON
Ingredients
•   300g of skinned salmon
•   Two teaspoons of olive oil
•   Two teaspoons of ground turmeric
•   ½ juice of a lemon
For celery
•   Two teaspoons of Olive oil
•   80g of finely chopped red onion
•   60g of tinned green lentils
•   Two finely chopped garlic cloves
•   2 cm fresh and finely chopped ginger
•   Two finely chopped Bird's eye chili
•   300g celery
•   Two teaspoons of mild curry powder
•   260g tomato

- 200ml chicken stock
- Two teaspoons of chopped parsley

Procedures
1.   Preheat your oven to 200°c and first. Then start preparing your spicy celery. Cut celery into 2 cm lengths.
2.   Place your fry pan on medium-low heat, then add the olive oil, onion, garlic, ginger, chili, and celery.
3.   Allow the ingredients to fry gently for 3 minutes. It should soften. Don't let it stay too long, so it doesn't turn brown.
4.   Then, add your curry powder and cook further for some minutes.
5.   Next, cut your tomatoes into eight wedges. Add the tomatoes, chicken stock, and lentils. Allow it simmer for 10 minutes.
6.   You can increase or decrease cooking time depending on how crunchy you want your celery.
7.   Mix your turmeric, oil, and lemon juice and rub the mixture on your salmon.
8.   Place the salmons on a tray and put in the oven to bake for 8-10 minutes.
9.   Garnish the celery with chopped parsley.
10.   Serve celery with salmon.

Nutritional Information
Servings: 2
Per serving:
Fats: 12g
Carbohydrates: 74mg
Protein: 2.9g
Calories: 612kcal

4.   CORONATION CHICKEN SALAD
Ingredients
- 300g of natural yogurt or low- fat yogurt
- One whole fresh lemon
- Two tablespoons of chopped coriander
- Two tablespoons of ground turmeric
- 400g of cooked chicken breast

- One tablespoon of mild curry powder
- 24 halves of finely chopped walnuts
- Four finely chopped dates
- 80g diced red onion
- 4 Bird's eye chili
- 160g Rocket to serve

Procedures

1. Squeeze out the lemon juice. Pick the seeds out thoroughly.
2. Mix the yogurt, lemon juice, and coriander in a bowl.
3. Then, add other spices, turmeric, walnuts, and chili.
4. Add the cooked chicken breast and onions. Stir the ingredients together properly.
5. Serve on rocket beds.
6. Other popular ingredients for making this special royal salad are mango chutney, almonds, or lemon zest.
7. You can add I teaspoon of mango chutney, I tablespoon of flaked almonds, and ½ lemon (zested and cut into smaller wedges)
8. You may also prefer to roast the red onions before putting them in the mixture.

Nutritional Information
Servings: 4
Per serving:
Fats: 21g
Carbohydrates: 53g
Protein: 34g
Calories: 559kcal

5. BAKED POTATOES WITH SPICY CHICKPEA STEW

Ingredients

- Six baking potatoes
- Two tins of 400g chickpeas (do not drain)
- Two tins 400g chopped tomatoes
- Two tablespoons of turmeric
- Two tablespoons of unsweetened cocoa powder
- Two teaspoons of chili flakes (You can use more or less depending on how spicy you like it)

- 2 cm grated ginger
- Four grated garlic cloves
- Two chopped red onions
- Two tablespoons of olive oil
- Two tablespoons of cumin seeds
- Two chopped yellow peppers (bite-sized)
- Two tablespoons of parsley
- A small splash of water
- Salt to taste.

Procedures

1. You should preheat your oven to 200°C first.
2. Put baking potatoes in the oven for 1 hour.
3. While the potatoes are baking, place your saucepan on medium heat. Add your olive oil and chopped onion. Cover the pan and let it cook for 5 minutes. Onions should not turn brown.
4. Then, add garlic, ginger, cumin, and chili. Allow the sauce to cook further on low heat.
5. Add turmeric and a little splash of water and let it cook more. Be careful and pay attention; don't let the saucepan get dry.
6. Now add tomatoes, cocoa powder, yellow pepper, and chickpea water.
7. Allow the sauce to boil together. When it boils, reduce the heat and let it simmer for 45 minutes or until it is thick.
8. You can add more salt and pepper if you please. Garnish the stew with parsley.
9. Ready to serve. Put the stew on top of the baked potatoes while serving.

Nutritional Information

Servings: 6

Per serving:

Fats: 11.4g

Carbohydrates: 72g

Protein: 2.5g

Calories: 481kcal

6. MELON AND GRAPE JUICE

Ingredients

- One cucumber
- 60g young spinach leaves
- 200g red grapes
- 200g cantaloupe melon

Procedures

1.   Wash melon, cucumber, grapefruits thoroughly. Wash all vegetables or fruits you wish to use as well.

2.   Remove seed from melon gently, peel off its skin, and cut melon into chunks.

3.   Peel off the skin from your cucumber, remove seeds, cut into halves and chop the cucumber roughly.

4.   Remove the stalks from your spinach leaves.

5.   Add ice cubes before blending if you please.

6.   Blend all the fruits and vegetables in a blender for not less than 30 seconds until it's smooth.

7.   Remove the excess foam from the surface of the blended juice.

8.   Add water to juice to make it thinner if you did not blend with ice.

9.   Put the juice in the refrigerator for a while to chill if you did not blend with ice. It is best served cold.

10.   Pour out the juice in separate glasses, serve.

11.   You may choose to use any other type of lemon. If you are using watermelon, you should remove the seeds and chop melon into smaller sizes before you blend.

12.   Instead of cucumber, you may prefer apples. Apples, grapes, and cantaloupe will go well with a handful of fresh mint. So if you are using apples, replace spinach leaves with mint for better taste.

NUTRITIONAL INFORMATION

Servings: 2

Per serving:

Fats: 0.4g

Carbohydrate: 14.4g

Protein: 0.7g

Calories 125kcal

7.   POLENTA BAKE

Ingredients

- One tablespoon of olive oil
- ½ diced medium-sized eggplant (if allergic, use mushrooms)
- ½ diced small sized zucchini
- ¼ teaspoon of salt
- ¼ cup of water
- ¼ teaspoon of freshly grounded pepper
- 5 ounces of baby spinach
- 1 cup of prepared marinara sauce
- ¼ cup of chopped fresh basil
- 7 ounces of prepared polenta
- 1 cup of shredded part-skim mozzarella
- Six tablespoons of cheese

Procedures

1. Preheat your oven to 232°c
2. Coat your baking dish with some cooking spray
3. Place a large nonstick skillet on medium-high heat.
4. Then add your diced eggplants, zucchini, salt, and pepper.
5. Allow the ingredients cook, but make sure you occasionally stir until the vegetables are soft and about to turn brown. This process should last 4-6 minutes. Don't let the vegetables burn.
6. Add your baby spinach. Let the spinach cook for about 3 minutes until it wilts. Stir only once.
7. Add your marinara sauce into the vegetables and stir. Let it heat for a minute or two,
8. Turn off the heat and stir in your basil.
9. Put polenta slices in your baking dish. Place them in a single layer. You can trim the slices to fit in the dish if necessary.
10. Sprinkle your cheese on the polenta
11. Top polenta with eggplant mixture. You can add more cheese.
12. Bake for 12-15 minutes until it's bubbling and the cheese has melted. Leave it for 5 minutes after baking before you serve.

Nutritional Information

Servings: 4

Per serving:
Fats: 2.7g
Carbohydrate: 4.4g
Protein: 4.11mg
Calories: 201kcal

8.   RAW CARROT AND ALMOND LOAF

Ingredients

- 6-8 medium-sized fresh carrots
- Juice of ½ medium-sized lemon
- ½ cup of almonds
- Fresh and chopped Parsley
- Four tablespoons of tahini
- 40g plain flour (optional)
- 30g Coconut sugar or as much as you wish (optional)
- ¼ teaspoon of baking powder (optional)

Procedures

- Grate your carrots properly
- Put the grated carrots in a food processor with an S blade.
- Blend carrots and lemon in the food processor. Let them whizz properly.
- Transfer the mixture into a bowl.
- Whizz up almond into the processor. Almonds must be well-grounded.
- Then, add the blended almonds and carrot mixture together.
- Add your parsley and tahini and blend them all.
- Transfer your mixture into a loaf thin. Put it in the oven to bake for some minutes.
- Cut into slices to serve. Serve as an appetizer.
- If you wish to add flour, sugar, and baking powder, you should cover the mixture with foil and leave it to bake for up to 45 minutes.
- Carrot and almond loaf can be served with cream cheese icing topping. But be careful; you don't want to take too much sugar.

• For cream cheese toppings, mix one tablespoon of low-fat yogurt, 20g cream cheese, lemon juice, and sugar in a bowl. Put it in a refrigerator to freeze. Then serve when the baked loaf is ready.

Nutritional Information

Servings: 4 slices

Per serving:

Fats: 7g

Carbohydrates: 30g

Protein: 6.5g

Calories: 103kcal

9.   BUCKET WHEAT PANCAKE

Ingredients

For pancakes

• 350ml of milk
• 150g of bucket wheat flour
• One tablespoon of olive oil
• One large egg

For your chocolate sauce

• 85ml of milk
• One tablespoon of double cream
• 100g of dark chocolates
• One tablespoon of olive oil
• 100g of chopped walnut
• 400g of hulled and chopped strawberries

Procedures

1.   First of all, make your pancake batter. Put milk, wheat, and egg into a blender. Make sure you blend well until it is smooth. Your mixture should not be too thick or runny.

2.   Heat frying pan until it smokes. Then add your olive oil.

3.   Pour batter into the frying pan to cover it completely. Make sure our pan is hot enough. One pancake should take only 1 minute.

4.   When you see it turning brown around the edges, flip it over with your spatula. Do this in one action so that the pancake doesn't break.

5.   Transfer into a plate when you are satisfied.

6.   The excess batter can be stored in your fridge for about five days in an airtight container. But you must mix well before you use it again.

7.   Next, prepare your chocolate sauce. Melt chocolate. You can do this easily by putting your chocolate in a heatproof bowl over a pan and simmering it in water.

8.   Mix melted chocolate in milk and whisk thoroughly. Add double cream and olive oil.

9.   Put strawberries on pancakes and roll-up.

10.   Spoon over chocolate sauce generously on the pancakes and sprinkle your chopped walnuts.

Nutritional Information
Servings: 6-8 pancakes
Per serving:
Fats: 9.9g
Carbohydrates: 81.2g
Protein: 16.8g
Calories: 455kcal

10.   KALE AND RED ONION DHAL WITH BUCKET WHEAT

Ingredients
- 160g of bucket wheat
- 100g of kale
- 200ml of water
- 160g of red lentils
- 400ml of coconut milk
- 2 cm of grated ginger cloves
- Two teaspoons of turmeric
- One seedless and finely chopped birds eye chili
- Three grated garlic cloves
- Two teaspoons of garam masala
- One sliced red onion

Procedures
- Place a deep saucepan on low heat. Add your olive oil and onions and allow it to cook for 5 minutes. Your onions should soften and not turn brown.

- Then, add your ginger, chili, and garlic. Be free to add as much chili as you wish, depending on how hot you like it. Allow it to cook for a minute more.
- Add turmeric, garam masala, and just a splash of water. Let it cook for another minute.
- Next, you add lentils, coconut milk, and 200ml of water. To get the right measurement for your water, you can just pour water into the coconut milk can and then into the pan.
- Mix your ingredients properly. Allow it to cook for 20 minutes more. If it becomes sticky, you can add a little more water.
- Then, add your kale, stir and cover it to cook for 5 minutes.
- Cook your buckwheat in a medium-sized saucepan separately for 10 minutes before curry is ready. You can do this 15minutes before the curry is ready.
- Serve bucket wheat and curry on a plate when they are ready.

Nutritional Information

Servings: 4

Per serving:

Fats: 12g

Carbohydrates: 72g

Proteins: 3.4g

Calories: 458kcal

11.   TUMERIC TEA

Ingredients

- One teaspoon of turmeric
- ½ teaspoon of cinnamon
- A pinch of black pepper
- ¼ teaspoon of ginger powder
- A pinch of cayenne pepper (optional)
- One teaspoon raw honey (optional)
- 2 cups of milk

Procedures

1.   Prepare your ingredients. You can use a tiny piece of peeled ginger roots instead of ginger powder.

2.	Blend all ingredients in a high-speed blender except the pepper. Make sure the ingredients are blended smoothly.
3.	You can use any milk of your choice, such as almond milk, pecan, dairy, coconut, or even bone broth.
4.	Be careful; turmeric tends to stain anything it touches. You should expect it to stain blender or countertops. You can use a thick paste of baking soda to wash off stains.
5.	Honey or maple syrup can be added to taste.
6.	Pour the mixture into a small saucepan and allow it heat for about 3-5 minutes. It should be hot and not boiling.
7.	Add your pepper as you desire and stir. You may choose to use black pepper, cayenne pepper, or both if you wish; it depends on how hot you want it.
8.	Serve hot and drink immediately.
Nutritional Information
Servings: 4
Per serving:
Fats: 4g
Carbohydrates: 4.4g
Protein: 1.9g
Calories: 61kcal

12.	DATE WITH WALNUTS CINNAMON BITES
Method 1
Ingredients
•	Six walnuts
•	Six pitted Medjool dates
•	Grounded cinnamon
Procedures
1.	Cut each walnut carefully into three slices
2.	Cut your dates also into three slices each.
3.	Then put a slice of walnut on each date.
4.	Dust the bite with cinnamon and serve.
Method 2
Ingredients
•	1 Ib of well-pitted Medjool dates
•	3/4 teaspoon of cinnamon
•	½ cup of ground walnuts
•	¼ teaspoon of salt

- ½ teaspoon of chia seeds
- ½ cup od almond meal
- One teaspoon of coconut oil

Procedures

1. Combine all ingredients except almond meal in a food processor. You can start with the dates only first to produce a better result. Whizz them until they come together in a ball.

2. Transfer them into a bowl. Roll the mixture together bit by bit into another bowl. You are free to roll into any size you please.

3. Put the balls in the freezer for 15 minutes. It will allow the ingredients to settle in properly and give you a better taste.

4. Roll the balls in the almond meal. Make sure the balls are well coated with almond meal.

5. Serve, and everyone takes a yummy bite.

Nutritional Information

Serving: 3-4

Per serving:

Fats: 8g

Carbohydrates: 21g

Protein: 2g

Calories: 168g

13. RED CHICORY, PEAR & HAZELNUT SALAD

Ingredients

- Two heads of red chicory
- Two red William pears
- A handful of rocket leaves
- Two tablespoons of hazelnut oil
- 25g of hazelnuts
- two tablespoons of mild salad oil
- one teaspoon of cider vinegar
- one teaspoon of green peppercorns (optional)

Procedures

1. Get your ingredients ready. You wash vegetables properly and observe other food hygiene.

2. Your hazelnuts should be toasted and chopped.

3. Cut out the chicory stalk carefully. Discard tired outer leaves. Arrange the leaves separately in 4 plates; you can make it 5-6 leaves per plate. They should not be too big.

4.   Take off the stalks from the pears. Make sure your pears are ripe. Cut them into four according to the length. Neatly cut out the cores of the pears and them into thin slices.

5.   Arrange your pears on top of the leaves.

6.   In a separate bowl, mix your dressing. Add oil and vinegar into the ball and salt to taste. If you wish to use peppercorns, crush them lightly in a bowl first before adding to the mix. Sherry is also a good option if you don't want to use vinegar.

7.   Spoon over half of your dressing on each salad plate.

8.   Then pour the remaining dressing on the rocket leaves separately. You can season with salt and pepper. Toss the leaves in the bowl.

9.   Pile the seasoned on top of each salad plate.

10.   Sprinkle your hazelnuts on the salad and serve.

Nutritional Information

Servings: 4

Per serving:

Fats: 15g

Carbohydrates: 8g

Protein: 2g

Calories: 176kcal

14.   KALE WITH LEMON TAHINI DRESSING

Ingredients

For your salad

- 250- 275g of curly kale
- one tablespoon of squeezed lemon juice
- ½ tablespoon of olive oil
- ½ tablespoon of toasted sesame oil
- one medium-sized carrot
- ½ tablespoon of pure maple syrup
- one medium-sized beet
- 2-3 tablespoons of pumpkin seeds.
- one tablespoon of hemp seeds (optional)
- A pinch of salt

For dressing

- three tablespoons of tahini
- one minced garlic clove

- three tablespoons of olive oil
- 80ml of squeezed lemon juice
- Salt and pepper

Procedures

1. Get your ingredients ready. Remove the large stems from the curly kale. You can use Tuscan kale if you wish.
2. Squeeze your lemon juice separately. Make sure you pick out all the seeds. Since you will need lemon juice for dressing, you should get more than one lemon.
3. Make sure your carrot and beet are peeled and grated.
4. Begin preparation. Pour your kale into a large salad bowl. Add lemon juice, oil, maple syrup, salt, and garlic.
5. Massage the mixture gently with your hand. Continue massaging until kale is soft and wilting. This process should last for 3-5 minutes.
6. Give kale extra time to soften by setting the mixture aside to marinate for 15-20 minutes.
7. Prepare your dressing. In a smaller bowl, add tahini, lemon juice, garlic, olive oil, salt, and pepper. Whisk the mixture properly. Taste and adjust seasoning as you desire. Then set aside.
8. When the kale is ready, pour the dressing over the kale. Toss the salad until it is evenly coated.
9. Add grated carrot and beet and toss it again until it has mixed well. If you are using hemp seeds, make sure they are hulled and sprinkle them over the salad.
10. Ready to serve

Nutritional Information

Servings: 6

Per serving:

Fats: 20g

Carbohydrates: 8g

Protein: 10g

Calories: 189kcal

15. BROCCOLI AND KALE GREEN SOUP

Ingredients

- 1 liter of stock
- one tablespoon of sunflower oil
- four sliced garlic cloves

- two thumb-sized ginger
- one teaspoon of ground coriander
- two pieces of fresh turmeric root or one teaspoon of ground turmeric
- ½ teaspoon of Himalayan salt
- 400g of roughly sliced courgettes
- 170g of broccoli
- 200g of chopped kale
- A pack of parsley for garnish; don't cut all
- two limes, zest, and juice

Procedures

1. Put your sunflower oil in a deep pan. Add garlic, coriander, ginger, turmeric, and salt. Then, fry for 2 minutes on medium heat. Stir so it doesn't burn.
2. Then add three tablespoons of water, so the spices don't get too dry,
3. Add courgettes and mix well. Make sure you mix the courgettes into the spices thoroughly. Allow it to coat well and cook for 3 minutes.
4. Add 400ml stock and allow it to simmer for 3 minutes. You can make stock by mixing two tablespoons of bouillon powder into boiling water.
5. Then, add your broccoli, lime juice, kale, and the remaining stock into the soup. Allow it to cook for 3-4 minutes. Your vegetables should cook until they soften.
6. Turn off the heat and add your roughly chopped parsley. Make sure you didn't chop all parsley. Leave some whole leaves for garnish.
7. Pour your soup into a blender and blend on high speed. Your soup should come out smooth, beautiful, and green.
8. Serve into four plates.
9. Garnish with zest lime and whole parsley.

Nutritional Information

Servings: 4

Per serving:

Fats: 8g

Carbohydrates: 14g

Protein: 10g

Calories: 182kcal

16.   Butter Bean and Vegetable Korma

Servings: 4

Butter bean and vegetable korma is a very nice dish that will catch your fancy. It is easy to make with bursts of traditional flavors that make it very delicious. You can get the whole meal cooked in less than an hour.

Ingredients
· three normal-size cloves of garlic
· one onion
· one fresh chili
· ½ piece of fresh ginger, thumb size
· 750g sweet potatoes
· one medium tomato
· 250g frozen peas
· 100g green sugar snaps/beans
· 2 tbsp. oil
· 400g large leek
· 400ml water
· one tin (400ml) coconut milk
· 3 tbsp. soy sauce/tamari
· 1 tbsp. honey
· 2 tsp. ground cumin
· Juice of a lemon
· 2 tsp. ground coriander
· 1 tsp. ground turmeric
· 2 tsp. salt
· 4 tsp. medium curry powder
· ½ tsp. freshly ground black pepper
· Bunch of fresh coriander
· one tin (400g) butterbeans

Procedures
1.   Put two tablespoons of oil into a large saucepan. Chop the tomato, red onion and put them into the pan

2.	Add the grated ginger, chili chopped garlic into the pan and have it cooked for about five minutes.
3.	Prepare the leeks and sweet potato. Do not forget to include the leafy bits (Also, remember to have the mixture in the pan stirred!)
4.	Add the ground cumin, curry powder, turmeric, ground coriander, and black pepper to the pan.
5.	Next, add 400 ml of water, one tin of coconut milk, two teaspoons of salt, the juice of 1 lemon, 1tablespoons of liquid sweetener, and three tablespoons of tamari (or soy sauce)
6.	Add the leeks, sweet potato, and beans and have the mixture stewed until the sweet potatoes are cooked or for about 20 minutes.
7.	Save a few peas for the purpose of garnishing and the rest of it inside. Also, add sugar snap peas. Serve!

17.	Trout with Roasted Vegetables
Servings: 4

Ingredients
•	one thinly sliced onion
•	two bell peppers, cubed and seeded
•	340 g (¾ lb.) Brussels sprouts, blanched and trimmed for seven minutes in boiling brine
•	30 ml (2 tbsp.) olive oil
•	11g (¼ cup) thinly sliced fresh basil
•	two trout fillets, with their skins (about 340 g or ¾ lb. each)
•	60ml (¼ cup) mayonnaise
•	Salt and pepper
•	30ml (2 tbsp.) water
Procedures
1.	Preheat the oven to 425°F (210°C) with the rack in the central position.
2.	Toss to coat the onion and bell peppers with the oil on a baking sheet that does not have a silicone mat or parchment paper. After then, place in the oven to bake for 15 minutes.

3.	Dive the Brussels sprouts into two equal halves and have them spread them onto the baking sheet. Include the peppers. Put the trout fillets in the middle of the vegetables—season with pepper and salt. Bake until the fish cook through and easily breaks apart with a fork or for a duration of about 10 minutes. Sprinkle with 30 ml (2 tablespoons) of the basil.
4.	Combine the rest of the basil (30ml/2 tbsp.), water, and mayonnaise in a bowl. Serve with the vegetables and trout.

18. Courgette tortilla

Servings: 2

Transform your day eggs into a flavor-packed dish with olives, peppers, and hummus - an outstanding and healthy lunch of vegetarian nature.

Ingredients
*	1 tbsp. olive oil
*	one large coarsely grated courgette
*	1 tsp. harissa
*	four large eggs
*	3 tbsps. reduced-fat hummus
*	one large red pepper, torn into strips
*	three pitted queen olives, quartered
*	Handful coriander

Procedures

1.	Heat the oil in a 20cm non-stick frying pan. Put the courgette and let it cook for some minute while stirring it periodically until it softens.
2.	Beat the eggs with the harissa and pour them into the pan.
3.	Proceed to cook gently. Stir to let the egg that is uncooked flow onto the base of the pan.

4.   When more than half has been cooked, do not touch it for about two minutes so that it will set. Place a plate, then take back to the pan, facing the uncooked part down, to have the cooking completed.

5.   Tip on top of a board and spread using the hummus to serve.

6.   Scatter with the coriander, olives, and pepper.

7.   Cut into quarters and eat cold or warm.

19. Lemon Paprika Chicken and Veggies

Servings: 6

This is a cool supper teeming with flavor. Lemon paprika chicken is snuggled in a bed of brussels sprouts and potatoes. You can get the whole dish prepared in half an hour's time.

Ingredients

- 6-8 bone-in chicken thighs
- 3 tbsp. olive oil
- Fresh ground pepper and salt, to taste
- 2 tsp. paprika
- 1 tsp. dried thyme
- Juice and zest of one lemon
- five divided garlic cloves
- 1 lb. baby potatoes
- 1 lb. brussels sprouts, halved and trimmed
- Pepper oil, salt, and olive (to taste)

Procedures

1. Mix together pepper, salt, olive oil, lemon zest, thyme, paprika, two minced garlic cloves, and lemon juice in a mixing bowl.

2. Pour all of these ingredients into a resealable bag and making sure that you evenly rub the mixture over all the chicken thighs. Place in the refrigerator for about hours.

3. Next, have your oven preheated to 230°C.

4. Cut and dice your vegetables and have them tossed into a bowl with pepper, salt, and olive oil (to taste).

5. Spread out the prepared vegetables on the pan on a parchment coated sheet pan. Take the chicken out from the fridge and make holes in the vegetables to nestle the chicken. Endeavor that you have everything kept in a layer for uniform cooking.

6. Place in the oven and bake for about 25-30 minutes. Set the oven to "broil" and have it broiled for 3-5 minutes on high, carefully watching to ensure the skin does not get burnt.

7. After then, allow the chicken to cool about for 5-10 minutes to retain juices and its full flavor.

20. Kale and Blackcurrant Smoothie

Servings: 2

Ingredients

- 1 cup freshly made green tea
- 2 tsp. honey
- one ripe banana
- ten baby kale leaves stalk removed
- six ice cubes
- 40g blackcurrants stalk removed and washed

Procedures

1. Stir in the honey in the green tea that you previously warm until it fully dissolves. Whiz together all the ingredients inside a blender, they become smooth. Proceed to serve instantly.

21. Buckwheat Pasta Salad

Servings: 1

Ingredients

- 50g buckwheat pasta (cooked the buckwheat in line with the packet instructions)
- Rocket, a large handful
- Basil leaves, a small handful
- 8 halved cherry tomatoes
- ten olives

- ½ diced avocado
- 20g pine nuts
- 1 tbsp. extra virgin olive oil

Procedures

1. With the exception of the pine nuts, gently mix all of the ingredients and set it in a bowl or on a plate, then proceed to scatter the pine over the top.

22. Miso Marinated Baked Cod with Stir-fried Greens and Sesame
Servings: 1

Ingredients:
- 20g (3½ tsp.) miso
- 1 tbsp. extra-virgin olive oil
- 200g (7-ounce) skinless cod fillet
- 20g (1/8 cup) sliced red onion
- 1 tbsp. mirin
- two finely chopped garlic cloves
- 40g (3/8 cup) sliced celery
- 1 tsp. finely chopped fresh ginger
- one finely chopped Thai chili
- 50g (¾ cup) roughly chopped kale
- 60g (3/8 cup) green beans
- 5g (2 tbsp.) parsley roughly chopped
- 1 tsp. sesame seeds
- 1 tbsp. tamari (or soy sauce, if not staying away from gluten)
- 1 tsp. ground turmeric
- 40g (¼ cup) buckwheat

Procedures

1. Combine one teaspoon of the oil, mirin, and miso. Rub on the cod and allow it to marinate for half an hour. Place in the oven and allow it to for 10 minutes at 230°C.

1.   Next, heat a large frying wok or pan with the rest of the oil. Put in the onion and have it stir-fried for a couple of minutes, then add the chili, garlic, celery, kale, green beans, and ginger. Fry and toss until the kale is cooked through and tender. There may be a need to pour a small amount of water into the pan to help in your cooking.

1.   Has the buckwheat cooked together with the turmeric in line with the package instruction?

1.   Add the tamari, parsley, and sesame seeds to the stir-fry. Serve with the fish and buckwheat.

23. Savory Truffles
Serving: 3
Ingredients
*   75g finely grated extra mature cheddar cheese
*   75g low-fat soft cheese
*   1 tbsp. paprika
*   1/3 of very finely chopped spring onion
*   1 tbsp. lightly toasted sesame seeds
*   2 tbsp. finely chopped fresh chives

Procedures
1.   Place the soft cheese inside a large mixing bowl. Mash it using a wooden spoon or a fork to make it soft.
2.   Add the spring onion and grated Cheddar, working it in until completely mixed. Season it with the ground pepper.
3.   Roll the mixture of the cheese into about ten small balls. Then, have some of them rolled into the paprika, some of them into the sesame seeds, and some of them into the chopped chives.
4.   Place in the refrigerator to chill. Serve.

24. Buckwheat Noodle and Green Bean Soup
Serving: 4
Ingredients
*   1 tsp. of toasted sesame oil

- 2 tbsp. of olive oil
- two spring onions of finely sliced
- 1 tsp. of finely sliced ginger root
- 1 liter of boiling water
- two carrots sliced into thin strips
- 1 tbsp. of tamari soy sauce
- 400g buckwheat noodles
- 125g (4 oz.) of frozen edamame beans
- 1 tbsp. of rice wine (this is optional)
- Pepper and salt
- Finely chopped fresh coriander

Procedures

1. Heat sesame oil and the olive in a large saucepan or wok. Stir in the carrots, spring onions, and ginger root and allow the resulting mixture to cook for some minutes.
2. Add one liter of boiling water into the mix. When it starts bubbling, include the tamari, noodles, edamame beans, and rice wine.
3. Then proceed to cook it until the vegetables and noodles cook through.
4. Take out from the heat and season with pepper and salt if desired, also garnish with coriander leaves. Serve.

25. Almond Butter and Alfalfa Wraps

Almond butter with a creamy consistency and alfalfa wraps coupled with some other ingredients all rolled up so you will have a wrap with low carbohydrates creating one of the tastiest and healthy snacks.

Servings: 1
Total time: 5 minutes

Ingredients
- Juice of 1 lemon
- 4 tbsp. of almond nut butter
- three finely sliced radishes

- 2-3 carrots grated
- 1 cup of alfalfa sprouts
- Nori sheets or lettuce leaves
- Pepper and salt

Procedures

1. Combine the almond butter with a sufficient amount of water and an ample amount of lemon juice so you will have a paste with your desired level of thickness.

1. Next, have the alfalfa sprouts and grated carrot mixed inside a bowl. Sprinkle with the remaining lemon juice that was set aside. Proceed to the season with pepper and salt to taste.
2. Using the almond butter, smear the nori sheets or lettuce leaves, depending on the one you are using. Top the resulting mixture with the alfalfa sprout mixture and carrot. Roll it up and serve. Enjoy!

26. Buckwheat Bean and Tomato Risotto
Servings: 4
Ingredients
- 2 tbsp. of butter or olive oil
- two cloves of chopped garlic
- eight ounces/225g buckwheat
- 400ml of vegetable stock or hot water
- eight ounces/225g broad beans
- ½ cup of sun-dried tomatoes inside an oil
- Juice of half a lemon
- 2 tbsp. of chopped coriander or basil
- two ounces/50g of toasted almonds
- Pepper and salt

Procedures

1. Heat the butter or olive oil inside a frying pan. Include the garlic and allow it to cook for a period of one minute.

2.   Next, place the buckwheat into the pan and have it stirred thoroughly. This is to allow the buckwheat to be coated in the oil.

3.   After that, add the stock or hot water. Then close the frying pan and let it simmer for 10 minutes.

4.   When you are done simmering, stir the broad beans in. Then proceed to cook until the beans are just tender, which should be for a few minutes.

5.   After that, add the fresh herbs, lemon juice, sun-dried tomatoes, and almonds. Season with pepper and salt to taste. Serve and enjoy your meal!

27. Chargrilled Beef, Onion rings, Red wine jus, Garlic Kale, and Roasted Potatoes

Ingredients

- 50gram of potatoes, peeled and cut into dice of 2cm
- 2g of parsley, nicely chopped
- 1 tbsp. of extra virgin olive oil
- 30g kale, sliced
- 30gram of red onion, sliced into rings
- Garlic
- Beef stock, 100ml
- 500–100g into a 2.3 cm-thick beef fillet steak
- 20ml red wine
- Half teaspoon of tomato puree
- Half teaspoon of cornflour, dissolved in 1 tablespoon of water

Procedures

1.   Get a saucepan to boil the potatoes for 6-7 minutes and drain.

2.   One teaspoon of oil will be added to the roasting pan. Roast till it's cooked over the oven. Preferably for 40-45 minutes.

3.   Replaced potatoes at every interval (10minutes) and removed after cooking.

4.   When done cooking, the chopped pieces of the parsley will be sprinkled and stirred thoroughly.

5.   Ingredients like the onions and butter will be fry over average heat for 10 minutes until the desirable result of been soft and uniquely caramelized is attained.

6.   Proceed to fry the garlic with oil (half-teaspoon) for 30-second, till it becomes soft but not golden.

7.   Place the kale and fry gently to soft for 1-minute.

8.   Heat saucepan till it begins smoking and coat the meat in half a teaspoon of oil over an average heat until meat is cooked or fried to your desired level.

9.   When the meat is cooked to an extent, remove it from the saucepan and keep safely to cool.

10.   To retain meat odors, add wine to a hot pan and allow bubbling to get the juice, with a strong concentration of flavor, before syrupy.

11.   The tomato, pure of the stock, will be added to cook pan to boil, following it, will be the cornflour that will be added in order to thicken its sauce.

12.   From the steak juice remaining, add some to serve with the kale, rings, onions, roasted potatoes, and red wine sauce to enjoy.

Nutritional Information:

Servings: 1

Nutrients per serving

Calories: 473 Fat: 2 g Carbohydrates: 12 g Protein: 12 g

28. Chocolate Cupcakes with Matcha Icing

Ingredients

- 300g self-rising flour
- ½ tsp vanilla extract
- 50ml vegetable oil
- two egg
- 200 ml of boiling water
- 400g caster sugar
- 120g cocoa
- 1 tsp salt
- 1 tsp fine espresso decaf coffee,
- 200ml milk
- For the icing:
- 1 tbsp matcha green tea powder

- ½ tsp vanilla bean paste
- 100g soft cream cheese
- 100 g butter, at room temperature
- 100 g icing sugar

Procedures
1. Preheat the oven, then line a cupcake tin with paper or silicone cake cases.
2. Mix the flour, sugar, cocoa, salt, and espresso powder in a large bowl
3. Add up the vegetable oil, milk, vanilla extract, and egg to the dry ingredients.
4. Use a mixer to beat the mix, then pour in the boiling water slowly until fully combined.
5. Spoon the batter evenly until the mixture bounces when tapped in between the cake cases
6. Cream the butter and icing sugar together to make the icing until it is soft and smooth.
7. Mix up with the vanilla and matcha powder and stir.
8. Add the cream cheese and beat until smooth.
9. Spread over the cakes.

Nutritional Information
Total Servings: 20
Per Serving
Calories: 150
Fat: 8 g
Carbohydrates: 16 g
Protein: 1 g
Fiber: 0 g

29. Kale, Edamame and Tofu curry
Ingredients
- ½ tbsp. rapeseed oil
- One large onion, chopped
- three cloves garlic, peeled and grated
- One large thumb (7cm) fresh ginger, peeled and grated
- One red chili, deseeded and thinly sliced
- ¼ tsp ground turmeric
- ¼ tsp cayenne pepper

- ½ tsp paprika
- ¼ tsp ground cumin
- ½ tsp salt
- 150g dried red lentils
- ½ -liter boiling water
- 30g frozen soya edamame beans
- 100g firm tofu, chopped into cubes
- a tomato, roughly chopped
- Juice of 1 lime
- 100g kale leaves stalk removed and torn

Procedures

1. Put the oil over low-medium heat in a heavy-bottom pan. Add the turmeric, cayenne, cumin, paprika, and oil. Remove and mix again before adding the red lentils.

2. Pour in the boiling water and cook for 10 minutes until the curry has a thick' porridge' consistency, then reduce the heat and cook for another 20-30 minutes.

3. Add soya beans, tofu, and tomatoes and continue to cook for another 5 minutes. Add the juice of lime and kale leaves and cook until the kale is tender.

Nutritional Information

Total Servings: 2

Per serving

Calories: 342

Fat: 5 g

Carbohydrates: 15 g

Protein: 28 g

30. Sesame Chicken Salad

Ingredients

- one tablespoon of sesame seeds
- one cucumber, peeled, deseeded, and sliced
- 100g baby kale, roughly chopped
- 60g pak choi, finely shredded
- ½ red onion, finely sliced
- 20g parsley, chopped
- 150g cooked chicken, shredded
- For the dressing:

- one tablespoon of extra virgin olive oil
- one teaspoon of sesame oil
- one lime
- one teaspoon of clear honey
- two teaspoons of soy sauce

Procedures

1. In a dry frying pan, put the sesame seeds and toast for 2 minutes to become lightly browned and fragrant. Put in a plate and set aside.

2. Put the olive oil, honey, soy sauce, sesame oil, and lime juice in a small bowl and mix to make the dressing.

3. Put in a large bowl, the kale, cucumber, pak choi, parsley, and red onion and gently mix. Pour the dressing into the mixture and continue mixing.

4. Share the salad on two plates topping them with the shredded chicken. Sprinkle the sesame seeds and serve.

Nutritional Information

Total Servings: 2

Per Serving

Calories 335

Fat 75

Cholesterol 74mg

Sodium 439mg

31. Sirt Food Mushroom Scramble Eggs

Ingredients

- two eggs
- 1 tsp ground turmeric
- 1 tsp mellow curry powder
- 20g kale, generally slashed
- 1 tsp additional virgin olive oil
- ½ superior bean stews, daintily cut
- Bunch of catch mushrooms, meagerly cut
- 5g parsley, finely slashed
- *optional* Add a seed blend as a topper and some Rooster Sauce to enhance

Procedures

1. Blend the turmeric and curry powder and include a little water until you have accomplished light glue.

2.   Steam the kale for 2–3 minutes.

3.   Warmth the oil in a skillet over medium heat and fry the bean stew and mushrooms for 2 to 3 minutes until they begin to darker and mollify.

4.   Include the eggs and flavor glue and cook over medium warmth at that point, add the kale and keep on cooking over medium heat for a further moment. At long last, include the parsley, blend well and serve.

Nutritional Information

Total Serving: 3

Per serving

Calories: 158 kcal

Protein: 9.96 g

Fat: 10.93 g

Carbohydrates: 5.04 g

32. Aromatic Chicken Breast, Kale, Red Onion, and Salsa

Ingredients

*   120g skinless, boneless chicken breast
*   two teaspoons ground turmeric
*   ¼ lemons
*   one tablespoon extra-virgin olive oil
*   50g kale, chopped
*   20g red onion, sliced
*   one teaspoon fresh ginger, chopped
*   50g buckwheat

Procedures

1.   To prepare the salsa, remove the tomato eye and finely chop. Add the chili, parsley, capers, lemon juice, and mix.

2.   Preheat the oven to 220°C. Pour one teaspoon of the turmeric, the lemon juice, and a little oil on the chicken breast and marinate. Allow staying for 5–10 minutes.

3.   Place an ovenproof frying pan on the heat and cook the marinated chicken for a minute on each side to achieve a pale golden color. Then transfer the pan containing the chicken to the oven and allow it to stay for 8–10 minutes or until it is done. Remove from the oven and cover with foil, set aside for 5 minutes before serving.

4.   Put the kale in a steamer and cook for 5 minutes. Pour oil into a pan and fry the red onions and the ginger to become soft but not colored. Add the cooked kale and continue to fry for another minute.

5.   Cook the buckwheat following the packet's instructions using the remaining turmeric.

6.   Serve alongside the chicken, salsa, and vegetables.

Nutritional Information

Total Serving: 3

Per serving

Calories 365

Fat: 11 g

Protein: 28 g

Fiber: 7 g

33. Smoked Salmon Omelette

Ingredients

- Two medium eggs
- 100 g Smoked salmon, cut
- 1/2 tsp Capers
- 10 g Rocket, slashed
- 1 tsp Parsley, slashed
- 1 tsp extra virgin olive oil

Procedures

1.   Split the eggs into a bowl and whisk well. Include the salmon, tricks, rocket, and parsley.

2.   Warm the olive oil in a non-stick skillet until hot yet not smoking.

3.   Include the egg blend and, utilizing a spatula or fish cut, move the mixture around the dish until it is even.

4.   Diminish the warmth and let the Omelettes cook through.

5.   Slide the spatula around the edges and move up or crease the Omelettes fifty-fifty to serve.

Nutritional Information

Total Serving: 2

Per serving

Calories: 148
Protein: 15.87 g
Fat: 8.73 g
Carbohydrates: 0.36 g

34. Green Salad Skewers
Ingredients
- Eight large black olives
- Eight cherry tomatoes
- One yellow pepper
- ½ red onion, chopped
- 100g cucumber, sliced
- 100g feta, chopped into 8
- Ingredients for the dressing
- two wooden skewers
- eight cherry tomatoes
- one tablespoon of extra virgin olive oil
- ½ lemons
- one teaspoon of balsamic vinegar
- ½ clove garlic, peeled and crushed
- Few basil leaves, finely chopped
- Few leaves oregano, finely chopped
- Salt
- Freshly ground black pepper

Procedures
1. Let the wooden skewers get soaked for 30 minutes with water
2. The skewers then need to be filled with the salad ingredients.
3. Mix all the dressing ingredients in a bowl, then pour over the skewers.

Nutritional Information
Total Serving: 2
Per serving
Calories 236
Fat 46g
Carbs 14g

Protein 7g

35. Citrus Fruit Salad
Ingredients
•	For Salad:
•	3 cups fresh kale, tough ribs removed and torn
•	one orange, peeled and segmented
•	one grapefruit, peeled and segmented
•	two tablespoons unsweetened dried cranberries
•	Dressing
•	two tablespoons extra-virgin olive oil
•	two tablespoons fresh orange juice
•	one teaspoon Dijon mustard
•	½ teaspoon raw honey
•	Salt and ground black pepper, as required
Procedures
1.	For the salad: in a salad bowl, place all ingredients and mix.
2.	For the dressing: place all ingredients in another bowl and beat until well combined.
3.	Place dressing on top of the salad and toss to coat well.
4.	Serve immediately.
Nutritional information
Total Serving: 2
Per serving
Calories 256
Total Fat 14.5g
Saturated Fat 2.1 g
Cholesterol 0 mg
Sodium 150 mg
Total Carbs 31.3 g
Fiber 4.8 g
Sugar 16.6 g
Protein 4.6 g
36. Tuscan Bean Stew
Ingredients
•	1 tbsp. extra virgin olive oil
•	50g red onion, finely sliced
•	30g carrot, stripped and finely sliced

- 30g celery, cut and finely sliced
- one garlic slice, finely sliced
- ½ 10,000 foot bean stew, finely sliced (optional)
- 1 tsp. Provence herbs
- 200ml vegetable stock
- 1 x 400g tin sliced Italian tomatoes
- 1 tsp. tomato puree
- 200g tinned blended beans
- 50g kale, generally sliced
- 1 tbsp. generally sliced parsley
- 40g buckwheat

Procedures

1.   Place the oil over low to medium heat in a medium saucepan and fry the onion, carrot, celery, garlic, chili (if used), and herbs gently until the onion is soft but not colorful.
2.   Stir in stock, tomatoes, and purée tomatoes and bring to boil. Attach the beans and allow cooking for 30 minutes.
3.   Add the kale and cook until tender for another 5–10 minutes, then add the parsley.
4.   Cook the buckwheat as instructed by the packet, drain and then serve with stew.
Nutritional Information
Total Serving: 2
Per serving
Calories 382
Fat: 2 g
Carbohydrates: 12 g
Protein: 12 g
Fiber: 0

37. Mocha chocolate Mosque
Ingredients
- Half cup of Water
- Two tablespoons of black coffee
- Dark chocolate, 15gram
- six egg white
- 3\4 cup of cream (heavy)

Procedures

1. Heat an averagely small amount of water and add the chocolate (15), two tablespoons of cocoa, and two tablespoon coffee boiler. NOTE the little amount of water is added to the button half of the boiler while the other will be added to the top half of the doubles boiler

2. Heat for 5-8 minutes, and stir the mixture gently until smooth.

3. Gently place the egg white into a bowl of an electric mixer balloon whip to whisk and gently add (2tbsp).

4. Next, gradually whip the recommended size of the heavy cup cream in stainless steel till it becomes solid and stiff; fold and add one- quarter of the egg white into a steamy chocolate mixture and fold the whipped cream gently in the remaining egg white and serve.

38. Strawberry Buckwheat Tabouleh

Ingredients

- Buckwheat 50gram
- Turmeric, one tablespoon
- Avocado, 80gram
- 20-gram. of Onions (Red)
- Medjool dates 25gram
- Capers, one tablespoon
- Parsley, 30gram
- 100gram of strawberries
- Extra virgin oil (1tbs)
- Lemon juice (half)
- 30gram of rocket

Procedures

1. Boil water over average heat.

2. And when heated, cook turmeric and buckwheat for eight minutes. (There is a need to go through the guide provided in the pack).

3. Remove water to dry and allow it to cool for a few minutes.

4.   Sliced/diced your tomatoes, avocado, and onions (red) parsley and capers smoothly and mix.
5.   Perfectly sliced the strawberries and mix with the salad alongside the lemon juice and oil.
6.   When this process is done, you serve, preferably on the rocket.
Servings: 1

39. Buckwheat Noodles with Chicken, Kale and Miso Dressing
Ingredients
•   Kale leaves, smoothly chopped (4-5 handful)
•   One- fifty (gram) of buckwheat noodles
•   Shitake mushrooms five sliced
•   One teaspoon of coconut
•   Smoothly diced brown onion (1)
•   One chicken breast (smoothly sliced)
•   One red chili, slicing should be thin and perfect
•   Two garlic cloves, preferably large and perfectly diced
•   Three tbsp. of tamari sauce
•   Organic miss, one, and half-table spoon
•   Virgin oil (1tbsp)
•   Lime juice (1tbsp)
Procedures
1.   Heat saucepan on an average heat to boiling water.
2.   Boil water to steam and add Kale in water to cook for a few minutes (4 minutes).
3.   When it's a bit wilted, remove the kales from boiled water and keep off.
4.   Buckwheat noddles should be added immediately to cook. (Promptly follow the guide on buckwheat pack).
5.   Thoroughly wash using cool water and set aside when done, mix the Shitake mushrooms in a small quantity of coconut oil to be fry for about four minutes till it's brown.
6.   Add a pinch of salt and keep aside.
7.
8.   With the sauce frying pan, the coconut will be heated over an average heat adding Ingredients the onion and chili to stir for 4 minutes before adding the chicken piece.

9.   When that is done, cook the meal for 4 minutes over average heat and stir.
10.   Also, add the quantity of water and the source with consistent stirring till chicken is cook to a desirable point.
11.   The kale and the soba noodles set aside will be added alongside the chicken to keep it spicy.
12.   Mix the drizzle and miso dressing and serve. Enjoy!

40. Aromatic Chicken Breast with Kale, Red Onions, Tomato, and Chili Salsa
Ingredients
*   A boneless and skinless chicken breast (250grams)
*   Four tablespoons of turmeric (ground)
*   Lemon juice (half)
*   Extra-virgin olive oil (2tbs)
*   Nicely chopped Kale (100 gram)
*   Nicely sliced onions (red), 40 gram
*   Two tablespoons of ginger freshly chopped
*   Buckwheat salsa 100gram
*   Tomatoes 260-gram (preferably two)
*   Bird-eye chili (2), nicely chopped
*   Nicely chopped parsley 10 gram
*   Two tablespoons of capers perfectly chopped
*   Half juice of a lemon
Procedures
1.   The tomato should be finely chopped, and the liquid should be kept in a safe place.
2.   The chili, parsley, lemon juice alongside the chopped tomato will be mixed.
3.   Heat over an average of 200°c.
4.   Put a little oil alongside the turmeric (1tbs), chicken breast, and lemon juice to cook for 8-10 minutes.
5.   Get a frying pan and heats until hot.
6.   Then, the immense chicken will be added and cooked for a minute or two (until it turns to gold).
7.   Send off to the oven, preferably on a baking tray, and cook for ten minutes.
8.   Remove from the baking tray and allow cooling for 3-5 minutes, then serving.

Servings: 2

41. Coronation Chicken Salad
Ingredients
•	One hundred and fifty grams of natural yogurt
•	Juice lemon (half).
•	One teaspoon of curry powder
•	Two teaspoons of coriander (perfectly chopped)
•	Ground turmeric (2tbs)
•	One hundred grams of cooked chicken breast (it must be cut into small sizes)
•	Twelve Walnuts, nicely chopped.
•	Nicely chopped Medjool dates (1)
•	Red Onions nicely diced (40g)
•	Bird-eye chili, (one)
•	Rocket to serve (80gram)

Procedures
1.	Place the yogurt, coriander, spices, and lemon juice in a bowl and mix.
2.	Other ingredients such as the walnuts halves, birds-eye, chili, and onions should be added.
3.	Serve preferably on a bed of rocket.

42. Baked Potatoes with Spicy Chickpea Stew
Ingredients
•	One red onion, nicely chopped
•	Two cloves- grated
•	Grated ginger (1cm)
•	One tablespoon, chili-flakes
•	Turmeric one -tablespoon
•	A sprinkle of water
•	Nicely chopped tomatoes (2×200g)
•	Cocoa powder (unsweetened) 1tbs
•	Two tin of chickpeas (200g each ×2)
•	Nicely chopped pepper in smaller sizes
•	Parsley with garnish (one tablespoon)
•	Salt
•	Pepper

Procedures
1.   Get all ingredients ready.
2.   Preheat oven, over an average heat/preferably 200 degree).
3.   When heated to a desired extent, place baking potatoes and cooked to your desired satisfaction, preferably for one hour: to fifteen minutes.
4.   Get a saucepan and placed in your olive oil alongside the chopped onion, and cooked till onions are soft.
5.   Cook more for five minutes over average heat, adding your garlic, chili, and ginger with it.
6.   Add water (a little splash), turmeric, and cook for some minutes (preferably 4-5 minutes).
7.   At this stage, the tomatoes, pepper, (yellow), and cocoa powder will be added and cooked for 35 minutes over an average heat till its sauce and thick to an extent.
8.   Add salt (a pinch of it), parsley (two tablespoons), and pepper (optional) when the stew is almost ready.
9.   Stir and serve on potatoes (Baked).

43. Cucumber, Pineapple, Parsley, And Lemon Smoothie
Ingredients
•   A bunch of leaf parsley nicely chopped.
•   Coconut water 3/4 cup.
•   Half cucumber, nicely chopped.
•   Two cups of frozen pineapple.
•   A drip of liquid stevia (5 drops preferably)
•   Ginger
Procedures
1.   Ensure the ingredients are ready.
2.   Get a blender, preferably a bigger blender.
3.   Place ingredients in one at a time to blend all.
4.   Blend ingredients over extremely high heat for three minutes till it's super creamy and smooth to serve.

44. Buckwheat Garden Salad
Ingredients
•   One cup of buckwheat

- Water, two cups
- Salt, half teaspoon
- Half cherrylotte nicely diced
- Green olives, 12 preferably large
- Two small nicely diced (yellow pepper)
- Smoothly chopped broccoli florets, one cup
- 50gram of walnuts, chopped
- Half cup of fresh dill, smoothly chopped
- One lime of juice
- Olive oil, one tablespoon
- Half teaspoon of black pepper

Procedures

1. Get a saucepan, medium-size, and fill with small water to boil.
2. Salt, buckwheat groats will be added to the boiling water to cook till it absorbed the ingredients.
3. Allow the cooked buckwheat to cool for an hour before adding green olive, cherrylotte, yellow bell pepper (diced), red onions, florets, chopped broccoli, and walnuts in a fitted bowl for thorough mixing.
4. Serve meal immediately after mixing or reserved for hours in a refrigerator.

Servings: 2

45. Bunless Beef and Burgers

Ingredients

- 30grams of red onions nicely chopped
- Two teaspoons of parsley smoothly chopped
- Sweet potatoes, 250grams
- Extra-virgin oil (2tbs)
- Two teaspoons of dried rose
- Two garlic cloves, sliced cheddar cheese, 10gram
- 150gram of red onions
- Tomato, 30gram, finely sliced
- Rocket 30g

Procedures

1. Firstly heat the oven to an average of 22°c.
2. We begin by peeling and slicing the potatoes into tiny thick chips.

3.   Mix the olive oil, garlic cloves, and rose will be tossed.

4.   Place tossed ingredients on a baking sheet to roast for 20-25 minutes.

5.   Next, the onions, parsley, and beef will be mix gently for minutes.

6.   Place oil over an average heated saucepan; add the olive oil to the saucepan.

7.   Place burger over one right side of the saucepan and place the onions rings at the left side, and cooked burger for seven minutes on each side of the pan, till it's desired results of been cooked well are meant.

8.   Onions ring should also be fried for two minutes or till it's well cooked.

9.   After cooking the burger, add cheese, red onions to cooked in over for 4-5 minutes.

10.   Remove from oven and top meal with rocket or tomato to serve with fries.

46. Strawberry Buckwheat Tabouleh

Ingredients

*   Buckwheat 50gram
*   Turmeric, one tablespoon
*   Avocado, 80gram
*   20-gram. of Onions (Red)
*   Medjool dates 25gram
*   Capers, one tablespoon
*   Parsley, 30gram
*   100gram of strawberries
*   Extra virgin oil (1tbs)
*   Lemon juice (half)
*   30gram of rocket

Procedure

1.   Boil water over average heat.

2.   And when heated, cook turmeric and buckwheat for eight minutes. (There is a need to go through the guide provided in the pack).

3.   Remove water to dry and allow it to cool for a few minutes.
4.   Sliced/diced your tomatoes, avocado, and onions (red) parsley and capers smoothly and mix.
5.   Perfectly sliced the strawberries and mix with the salad alongside the lemon juice and oil.
6.   When this process is done, you serve, preferably on the rocket.
Servings: 1

47. Buckwheat Noodles with Chicken, Kale and Miso Dressing

Ingredients
- Kale leaves, smoothly chopped (4-5 handful)
- One- fifty (gram) of buckwheat noodles
- Shitake mushrooms five sliced
- One teaspoon of coconut
- Smoothly diced brown onion (1).
- One chicken breast (smoothly sliced)
- One red chili, slicing should be thin and perfect
- Two garlic cloves, preferably large and perfectly diced
- Three tbsp. of tamari sauce
- Organic miss, one, and half-table spoon
- Virgin oil (1tbsp)
- Lime juice (1tbsp)

Procedures
1.   Heat saucepan on an average heat to boiling water.
2.   Boil water to steam and add Kale in water to cook for a few minutes (4 minutes).
3.   When it's a bit wilted, remove the kales from boiled water and keep off.
4.   Buckwheat noddles should be added immediately to cook. (Promptly follow the guide on buckwheat pack).
5.   Thoroughly wash using cool water and set aside when done, mix the Shitake mushrooms in a small quantity of coconut oil to be fry for about four minutes till it's brown.
6.   Add a pinch of salt and keep aside.

7. With the sauce frying pan, the coconut will be heated over an average heat adding Ingredients the onion and chili to stir for 4 minutes before adding the chicken piece.

8. When that is done, cook the meal for 4 minutes over average heat and stir.

9. Also, add the quantity of water and the source with consistent stirring till chicken is cook to a desirable point.

10. The kale and the soba noodles set aside will be added alongside the chicken to keep it spicy.

11. Mix the drizzle and miso dressing and serve. Enjoy!

48. Aromatic Chicken Breast with Kale, Red Onions, Tomato, and Chili Salsa

Ingredients

- A boneless and skinless chicken breast (250grams)
- Four tablespoons of turmeric (ground).
- Lemon juice (half).
- Extra-virgin olive oil (2tbs)
- Nicely chopped Kale (100 gram)
- Nicely sliced onions (red), 40 gram
- Two tablespoons of ginger freshly chopped
- Buckwheat salsa 100gram
- Tomatoes 260-gram (preferably two).
- Bird-eye chili (2), nicely chopped
- Nicely chopped parsley 10 gram
- Two tablespoons of capers perfectly chopped
- Half juice of a lemon

Procedures

1. The tomato should be finely chopped, and the liquid should be kept in a safe place.

2. The chili, parsley, lemon juice alongside the chopped tomato will be mixed.

3. Heat over an average of 200°c.

4. Put a little oil alongside the turmeric (1tbs), chicken breast, and lemon juice to cook for 8-10 minutes.

5. Get a frying pan and heats until hot.

6. Then, the immense chicken will be added and cooked for a minute or two (until it turns to gold).

7.	Send off to the oven, preferably on a baking tray, and cook for ten minutes.
8.	Remove from the baking tray and allow cooling for 3-5 minutes, then serving.
Servings: 2

49. Coronation Chicken Salad
Ingredients
•	One hundred and fifty grams of natural yogurt
•	Juice lemon (half).
•	One teaspoon of curry powder.
•	Two teaspoons of coriander (perfectly chopped)
•	Ground turmeric (2tbs).
•	One hundred grams of cooked chicken breast (it must be cut into small sizes)
•	Twelve Walnuts, nicely chopped.
•	Nicely chopped Medjool dates (1)
•	Red Onions nicely diced (40g)
•	Bird-eye chili, (one)
•	Rocket to serve (80gram)

Procedures
1.	Place the yogurt, coriander, spices, and lemon juice in a bowl and mix.
2.	Other ingredients such as the walnuts halves, birds-eye, chili, and onions should be added.
3.	Serve preferably on a bed of rocket.

50. Baked Potatoes with Spicy Chickpea Stew
Ingredients
•	One red onion, nicely chopped
•	Two cloves- grated
•	Grated ginger (1cm)
•	One tablespoon, chili-flakes
•	Turmeric one -tablespoon
•	A sprinkle of water
•	Nicely chopped tomatoes (2×200g)
•	Cocoa powder (unsweetened) 1tbs

- Two tin of chickpeas (200g each ×2)
- Nicely chopped pepper in smaller sizes
- Parsley with garnish (one tablespoon)
- Salt
- Pepper

Procedures

1. Get all ingredients ready.
2. Preheat oven, over an average heat/preferably 200 degree).
3. When heated to a desired extent, place baking potatoes and cooked to your desired satisfaction, preferably for one hour: to fifteen minutes.
4. Get a saucepan and placed in your olive oil alongside the chopped onion, and cooked till onions are soft.
5. Cook more for five minutes over average heat, adding your garlic, chili, and ginger with it.
6. Add water (a little splash), turmeric, and cook for some minutes (preferably 4-5 minutes).
7. At this stage, the tomatoes, pepper, (yellow), and cocoa powder will be added and cooked for 35 minutes over an average heat till its sauce and thick to an extent.
8. Add salt (a pinch of it), parsley (two tablespoons), and pepper (optional) when the stew is almost ready.
9. Stir and serve on potatoes (Baked).

51. Cucumber, Pineapple, Parsley, And Lemon Smoothie

Ingredients

- A bunch of leaf parsley nicely chopped.
- Coconut water 3/4 cup.
- Half cucumber, nicely chopped.
- Two cups of frozen pineapple.
- A drip of liquid stevia (5 drops preferably)
- Ginger.

Procedures

1. Ensure the ingredients are ready.
2. Get a blender, preferably a bigger blender.
3. Place ingredients in one at a time to blend all.

4.   Blend ingredients over extremely high heat for three minutes till it's super creamy and smooth to serve.

52. Buckwheat Garden Salad
Ingredients
*   One cup of buckwheat
*   Water, two cups
*   Salt, half teaspoon
*   Half cherrylotte nicely diced
*   Green olives, 12 preferably large
*   Two small nicely diced (yellow pepper)
*   Smoothly chopped broccoli florets, one cup
*   50gram of walnuts, chopped
*   Half cup of fresh dill, smoothly chopped
*   One lime of juice
*   Olive oil, one tablespoon
*   Half teaspoon of black pepper
Procedures
1.   Get a saucepan, medium-size, and fill with small water to boil.
2.   Salt, buckwheat groats will be added to the boiling water to cook till it absorbed the ingredients.
3.   Allow the cooked buckwheat to cool for an hour before adding green olive, cherrylotte, yellow bell pepper (diced), red onions, florets, chopped broccoli, and walnuts in a fitted bowl for thorough mixing.
4.   Serve meal immediately after mixing or reserved for hours in a refrigerator.
Servings: 2

53. Bunless Beef and Burgers
Ingredients
*   30grams of red onions nicely chopped.
*   Two teaspoons of parsley were smoothly chopped.
*   Sweet potatoes, 250grams
*   Extra-virgin oil (2tbs)
*   Two teaspoons of dried rose
*   Two garlic cloves, sliced cheddar cheese, 10gram
*   150gram of red onions

- Tomato, 30gram, finely sliced.
- Rocket 30g.

Procedures

1. Firstly heat the oven to an average of 22°c.
2. We begin by peeling and slicing the potatoes into tiny thick chips.
3. Mix the olive oil, garlic cloves, and rose will be tossed.
4. Place tossed ingredients on a baking sheet to roast for 20-25 minutes.
5. Next, the onions, parsley, and beef will be mix gently for minutes.
6. Place oil over an average heated saucepan; add the olive oil to the saucepan.
7. Place burger over one right side of the saucepan and place the onions rings at the left side, and cooked burger for seven minutes on each side of the pan, till it's desired results of been cooked well are meant.
8. Onions ring should also be fried for two minutes or till it's well cooked.
9. After cooking the burger, add cheese, red onions to cooked in over for 4-5 minutes.
10. Remove from oven and top meal with rocket or tomato to serve with fries.

54. BLACKCURRANT AND RASPBERRY JELLY

Raspberry and Blackcurrant Jelly is a flavor-filled formula that's easy to whip up. This lovely recipe uses fresh fruits, and it's ideal for preserving your raspberries and blackcurrants.

Ingredients

- 600g Mixed fresh fruits, i.e., raspberries and blackcurrants
- 0.5ml Lemon juice, freshly squeezed
- 300 ml Water
- 100g Clear or 'runny' honey
- 10g Gelatine

Procedures

1.   Put the fresh berries in a clean dish. Add the fresh lemon juice, honey, and water and bring the mixture to a delicate stew for about 10 minutes.

Allow the mixture to cool a bit and strain the juice through a fine-mesh strainer into a bowl. Remove the seeds from the berries as much as you can. To squeeze the remaining juice, gently mash the residue on the strainer.

1.   Break the gelatine into little bits and mix it with some warm water for two minutes in a little bowl to dissolve. As you drop the gelatine into the juice, pull it apart and mix it in well until the whole mixture is uniform. Prepare your jelly molds and pour the gelatine-juice mixture in. Another option is to leave the mixture to set in the bowl. Ideally, you should allow it to set in a cool place before serving, preferably your fridge.

2.   To make it easier to remove the jelly, dip the jelly molds into hot water for some seconds once the jelly is set. Turn out the jelly on a plate before serving.

Serve as a mouthwatering summer pudding.

55. GREEN TEA SMOOTHIE

This delicious green tea smoothie—thanks to a bit of honey—is filled with grapes, spinach, green tea, and avocado. And, of course, it's a low-carb vegan recipe packed with all-natural, all-good ingredients.

Ingredients

•   3 cups White grapes, frozen
•   2 cups fresh baby spinach leaves, washed
•   1½ cups Green tea, strongly brewed (see note below) and cooled
•   1 Avocado, slightly ripe
•   2 tsp Honey

Procedures

1.   Add the baby spinach, grapes, green tea, avocado, and honey in a blender; blend well until smooth. Serve right away.

2.   Note: To brew green tea with a strong taste, use double the quantity of tea (or two bags); don't steep it for too long, though. Leave the green tea bag to infuse for about three minutes. Anything more than that, and you'll end up with over-brewed, bitter tea.

56. APPLE PANCAKES WITH BLACKCURRANT COMPOTE
Ingredients
•   75g Rolled oats
•   125g White flour
•   One teaspoon Baking powder
•   Two tablespoons Castor sugar
•   A pinch of salt
•   2 Apples, cored, peeled, and finely chopped
•   300ml Semi-skimmed milk
•   2 Egg whites
•   Two teaspoons Extra-light olive oil
•   Ingredients for compote: 120g blackcurrants, washed and followed expelled; 2 tablespoons castor sugar, and three tablespoons water.
Procedures
1.   To prepare the blackcurrant compote, add the blackcurrants, water, and sugar in a saucepan. Let it simmer for 10-15 minutes. In a big bowl, thoroughly mix the flour, oats, baking powder, sugar, and salt to make the pancake batter. Mix in the apple and afterward add in the milk little-by-little, whisking until the whole mixture is smooth. Stiffly beat the egg whites and fold into the batter. Pour the batter into a jug.
2.   Heat 1/2 teaspoon oil in a Teflon pan on medium-high heat and pour in about 1/4 of the batter. Cook the pancakes on both sides till they're golden brown. Wipe the pan and repeat the above process to get four servings.
3.   Serve the pancakes with the compote dribbled over.

57. BRAISED PUY LENTILS
Ingredients
•   300g Puy lentils, rinsed
•   One small onion, finely chopped
•   2 Celery stalks, finely diced

- 1 Carrot, diced
- Three tablespoons Extra-virgin olive oil
- 3 Thyme twigs, fresh
- 750ml Hot vegetable stock, from a first-rate cube
- Lemon juice, freshly squeezed
- Extra-virgin olive oil, to taste

Procedures

1. Heat the oil over medium heat in a wide pan. Add the onion, celery, and carrot and cook for some minutes, stirring until the onion softens.

2. Stir in the lentils to coat them in the oil, then add the thyme and hot stock—season with freshly ground black pepper. Bring to the boil, then cook on low heat. Let the lentils simmer for 15-20 minutes, or until they are soft enough to fully absorb the stock.

3. Add some boiling water if the lentils seem dry. Remove the thyme and add the lemon juice. To the lentils, pour in a good amount of olive oil and check the seasoning. Serve alongside some tasty pork sausages at your desired temperature.

58. CHINESE-STYLE PORK AND PORK CHOP

Ingredients

- 4 Pork chops
- One tablespoon Soy sauce
- One tablespoon Rice wine
- Two teaspoons Sugar
- 1/2 teaspoon salt
- One pinch Pepper (or five-spice powder)
- One tablespoon Crushed garlic
- 1 Egg
- Six tablespoon Cornstarch
- Cooking oil

Procedures

1. Use a meat hammer to pound the pork, so it's really tender. In case you're wondering about the exact thickness, pound, so it's just about a quarter-inch thickness. Let it marinate for about 30 minutes. (You should marinate for no less than ten minutes, up to a day).

2.	Before you start frying, pour cornstarch into pork marinade and mix thoroughly.
3.	Heat the oil in a wide skillet, enough to cover its base. Place the pork in oil when it starts to simmer—Cook pork chops over medium-high heat until properly cooked.

59. SALMOND SIRT SUPER SALAD
Ingredients
*	50g Arugula (aka salad rocket)
*	50g Chicory leaves
*	100g Smoked salmon cuts
*	80g Avocado, peeled, cored, and sliced
*	15g Walnuts, chopped
*	One tablespoon Capers
*	One large Medjool date, hollowed and chopped
*	One tablespoon Extra-virgin olive oil
*	Juice of a quarter lemon
*	10g parsley, finely chopped
*	50g Celery, sliced with leaves
*	20g Red onion, chopped

Procedures
1.	Arrange the salad leaves in a bowl or plate. Mix the rest of the ingredients and pour the mixture on the leaves.
2.	For a lentil sirt super salad, substitute the smoked salmon for 100g canned green lentils or cooked Puy lentils.
3.	For a chicken shirt super salad, replace the salmon with cooked chicken breast cutlets.
4.	For a fish sirt super salad, replace the smoked salmon with canned fish.

60. SKEWERS WITH SATAY PEANUT SAUCE
Ingredients
*	500g beef
*	two cloves of garlic, crushed
*	1/2 Onion, finely chopped (can be replaced with red, white, or spring onions)
*	one red chili, minced and seeds removed
*	one tablespoon Ginger, finely ground

- one lime, zested
- two tablespoons Soy sauce
- two tablespoons Brown sugar
- Cilantro
- Cut lime, optional
- Rice, optional
- Prawn crackers, optional

Ingredients for the sauce
- 200g Peanuts, crushed
- 1/2 Red onion, finely chopped
- two tablespoons Brown sucrose sugar
- three cloves of garlic, crushed
- 1/2 tablespoon ginger, finely chopped
- two red chilies, deseeded and minced
- 50ml Coconut milk
- two tablespoon Soy sauce
- 1 Lemon, freshly squeezed

Procedures

1.   Before threading, soak wooden or bamboo skewers in cold water for about half an hour to keep them from burning up.

2.   Cut the beef into long slices (about a quarter-inch thick). Mix the sugar, ginger, garlic, chili, onion, lime zest, and soy sauce. Stir in the beef, cover, and marinate for about 30 minutes (maximum of 12 hours). Once it is marinated, fix the beef on wooden skewers and place them on a tray. Set aside the marinade.

3.   To prepare the satay sauce, add the crushed peanuts, sugar, and onion in a wide frying pan, cooking over medium heat for about 5 minutes. Keep stirring until all the sugar has melted. Raise the heat, cook till peanuts are golden-brown, and then add the spices. After around a minute, add the water, coconut milk, and soy sauce. Boil the mixture over little heat and stir every now and then until thick (or about 15 minutes). Mix in the lemon juice and add seasoning to taste. Blend the mixture to a thick paste.

4.   Heat up a dry griddle on high heat (or you can preheat a grill to medium). Bring the beef skewers to the griddle, cooking for a couple of minutes. Brush each side with leftover marinade from time to time until they start charring at the ends. Dress with cilantro leaves and serve with rice salad, cut lime, or prawn crackers, as you'd like.

61. ASIAN SHRIMPS STIR-FRY WITH BUCKWHEAT NOODLES

Ingredients
*   150g raw jumbo shrimp, shelled and deveined
*   two teaspoons Tamari (soy sauce is also fine if you're not staying away from gluten)
*   two teaspoons Extra-virgin olive oil
*   75g Soba (aka buckwheat noodles)
*   two cloves of garlic, finely chopped
*   1 Thai chili, finely chopped
*   One teaspoon fresh ginger, finely minced
*   20g Red onions, sliced
*   45g Celery, trimmed and sliced, with leaves reserved
*   75g Green beans, minced
*   50g Kale, coarsely chopped
*   100ml Chicken stock
*   5g Celery (or lovage) leaves

Procedures
1.   Heat a frying pan and cook shrimps in tamari and olive oil (1 teaspoon each) for about 2-3 minutes.
2.   Turn the shrimps onto a plate. Clean the pan with a paper towel, as you'll be using it again.
3.   Boil the noodles in water for 5–8 minutes, or as required on the packaging. Drain well in a colander and set aside.
4.   Fry the onions, chili, ginger, green beans, celery, and kale in the leftover oil and tamari over medium-high heat for 2–3 minutes. Add the chicken stock and let it boil. Next, leave it to simmer for about 1-2 minutes until the vegetables are cooked but still crunchy.

5.   Add the celery leaves, shrimp, and noodles to the frying pan, boil and then let it cool down before serving.

62. BUCKWHEAT FRUIT AND NUT LOAF

Ingredients
- 1 cup Buckwheat flour
- 1 cup Nuts (pecans, walnuts, almonds, as you'd like)
- One tablespoon Baking soda
- One tablespoon Baking powder
- One tablespoon Cinnamon
- A pinch of salt
- 1½ Dried fruits (raisins, dried plums, apricots, dates, and figs)
- 110g Seeds (pumpkin, sunflower, sesame, or hemp seeds) (1/2 cup)
- Two tablespoons Sugar syrup or coconut sugar (optional)
- 295ml Water or more, as needed
- 60ml Oil

Procedures
1.   Preheat your oven to 180C. Grease a bread pan and line it with a sheet of waxed paper. Mix the baking powder, baking soda, salt, and cinnamon into the flour.
2.   Chop the dried fruit and nuts and pour in the flour blend alongside the seeds.
3.   Add oil and water to the mix and mix thoroughly with a spoon. Pour the dough into the greased pan and sprinkle with seeds (oatmeal is also fine).
4.   Bake for 30 minutes or until a toothpick comes out clean.

63. SHAKSHUKA WITH FETA

Ingredients
- three tablespoons Extra-virgin olive oil
- 1 Large onion, sliced thinly
- One large Red bell pepper, seeded and thinly sliced
- three cloves of garlic cloves, thinly sliced
- One teaspoon Cumin

- One teaspoon Smoked paprika
- 1/8 teaspoon ground cayenne, or to taste
- A dash of coriander
- 2-3 (28 oz) Whole tomatoes, peeled and coarsely chopped
- 3/4 teaspoon Kosher salt, to taste
- 1/4 teaspoon Black pepper, to taste
- 5 oz Feta cheese, crumbled
- 6 Eggs
- Chopped parsley, for serving
- Hot sauce, for serving

Procedures

1. Preheat the oven to 375 degrees. Sauté the onions, garlic, and bell pepper in simmering olive oil in a large, oven-safe skillet. Cook over medium-low heat for about 20 minutes until the onions are tender. Immediately, stir in the cumin, paprika, coriander, and cayenne pepper, and cook for a minute. Next, add in the tomatoes and season with salt and pepper to taste; simmer the mixture for about 10 minutes. Taste and add more salt and pepper to taste. Sprinkle a good amount of the crumbled cheese on the skillet.

2. Using the back of a spoon, form craters and crack eggs into them. Season eggs with salt and pepper. Transfer skillet to oven and bake for roughly 7 to 10 minutes until egg whites set. Sprinkle with chopped parsley and serve with hot sauce.

64. VANILLA AND CHOCOLATE SANDWICH REFRIGERATOR COOKIES

Ingredients

- 1½ cups Butter
- 1⅓ cups Sugar, preferably powdered
- One teaspoon Vanilla
- 1/4 teaspoon salt
- 2⅔ cups Pastry flour
- 1/2 cup Powdered cocoa
- One teaspoon Baking powder

Ingredients for filling

- 1⅓ cups Sugar, also powdered
- 1/2 cup butter
- One teaspoon Vanilla
- 1 Egg white or 1/4 cup meringue powder
- Water, as needed

Procedures

1. Cream the butter, sugar, and salt with a mixing paddle or flat paddle attachment of your stand mixer until light. Next, add the vanilla to the butter mixture. Stir the flour, cocoa, and baking powder together in a separate bowl.

2. Pour the flour mix into the butter mixture and beat until thoroughly mixed. You can also work the dough with your hands on a clean counter. For best results, you should aim for a clay-like texture.

3. While you mix in the dough, it will be crumbly at first. As the butter gets soft, the dough moistens and clumps into a firm ass; you can easily mold with your hands.

4. Roll the dough on the counter with your hands to form a long round log measuring around 1½ by 20 inches. If you'd prefer neat, circular cookies, roll the dough into a round, uniform shape. In case the dough is too soft to cut or form, refrigerate it for a while.

5. While the dough is still cold and firm, cut it into quarter-inch slices with a serrated knife. Use a ruler if you prefer uniform thickness. Roll the log a quarter turn after cutting a few cookies to keep it around. If cookies have a flat edge, keep the edges rounded with your fingers before baking.

6. Heat up the oven to 350 degrees. Place cookies on a thinly buttered baking pan and bake for about 12 minutes or until cookies are puffed and not glossy. Place cookies on a wire tray to cool.

7. To prepare the filling, beat the butter in a small bowl until smooth and fluffy. Add the vanilla and sugar. Stir in the egg white or meringue powder to make the filling solid, and beat until smooth. To make sandwich cookies, put a little amount of filling on a cookie and press another cookie to the filling, back to back. Repeat with the rest of the cookies. Allow the filling to set before serving cookies. Store in a cool place.

8.   Cookie dough can be refrigerated for up to 2 weeks or frozen for a couple of months. With refrigerator cookies, you can always bake as needed, whenever you want.

65. MOONG DAL TADKA

Ingredients
- 1/2 cup Moong dal (husked, split mung lentils)
- One medium onion, finely chopped
- One medium tomato, chopped
- 1/2 inch Ginger, grated
- 1/4 teaspoon Red chili powder (or cayenne pepper)
- 1/3 teaspoon Turmeric powder
- 1½ cups water
- Salt, as needed

Ingredients for tempering
- One teaspoon Cumin seeds
- 4-5 cloves of garlic, lightly crushed
- 1/4 teaspoon Red chili powder (or cayenne pepper)
- 1/4 or 1/2 teaspoon Garam masala powder
- 1-2 green chili, sliced
- A dash of hing (optional)

2-3 tablespoons oil or butter

Procedures

1.   Wash moong dal in water. Add finely chopped onions, tomatoes, and ginger to a pressure cooker. Next, add in turmeric powder and red chili powder. Add 1½ cups of water to the mixture and stir properly.

2.   Cook the dal for 5 to 6 whistles on medium heat until it's soft. Depressurize the cooker and stir the dal. If it looks thick, add more water and let it simmer for a minute or two till you get the desired thickness. Add salt as needed and mix properly. Set dal aside.

3.   Measure and prepare all ingredients required for tempering. Heat 2 to 3 tablespoons oil or butter in a pan, add one teaspoon cumin seeds. Fry the cumin seeds on low to medium-low heat so they don't get burnt. The cumin seeds should change shading and pop.

4.   Once you see a change in color, add crushed garlic cloves and sliced green chilies—Fry for a few seconds. Try not to brown the garlic. Next, add garam masala powder, chili powder, and a dash of hing. Turn off the heat, so the added spices don't get burnt.

5.   Mix the spice blend thoroughly with a spoon while you pour the tempering in the moong dal. Stir the moong dal, and you're all set!

6.   Moong Dal Tadka is best served hot with steamed basmati rice. Garnish with coriander leaves, as you'd like. Add a little bit of lemon juice for a tangy meal.

66. GRILLED MACKEREL WITH TOMATOES AND STEAMED VEGETABLE

Ingredients

- 2 Sweet potatoes, chopped
- 2 Leeks, chopped
- 150ml Vegetable stock
- One tablespoon Olive oil
- 300g mackerel fillets
- 200g cherry tomatoes, on the vine
- 50g Black olives pitted
- 1 Lemon

Procedures

1.   Preheat the oven to 200C. Add potatoes and leeks into a roasting pan. Pour the vegetable stock over, then sprinkle with one tablespoon olive oil. Season to taste and roast for 15-20 minutes.

2.   Next, add mackerel fillets, cherry tomatoes, and olives to the pan. Add freshly squeezed juice from 1 lemon over.

3.   Roast for 10 minutes more or until mackerel is cooked through and tomatoes are soft.

67. POMEGRANATE QUINOA PILAF

Ingredients

- Two tablespoons Olive oil (you can use butter or vegetable oil)
- 1/2 medium onion, chopped
- 1 cup Quinoa

- 2 cups Chicken broth, low-sodium (you can use stock or water)
- 1/2 cup Pomegranate seeds
- 1/2 cup Scallions, diagonally sliced
- One tablespoon Flat-leaf parsley, freshly chopped
- Juice of 1/2 Lemon
- One teaspoon fresh Lemon zest
- One teaspoon Sugar
- Salt
- Black pepper, freshly ground
- 1/2 cup Slivered almonds, toasted

Procedures

1. Heat 1 tablespoon olive oil in a large pot over medium-high heat. Sauté the onions until translucent and fragrant. Add the quinoa and stir, so it's coated. Add the chicken broth and leave it to boil. Turn the heat down and simmer for around 20 minutes, until broth is absorbed and the quinoa is soft.

2. In a big bowl, add the remaining olive oil, pomegranate seeds, scallions, chopped parsley, lemon zest and juice, and sugar. Add the quinoa and season with salt and pepper to taste. Garnish with toasted, fragmented almonds.

68. BANANA, DATE AND WALNUT PORRIDGE

Ingredients

- 80g Rolled oats
- 50g Dried dates, chopped
- 20g Walnuts, chopped
- 570ml water
- One medium banana, sliced

Procedures

1. Place walnuts, dates, and oats in a small microwave-safe bowl with a cup of a cup water. Microwave on high for 1½ minutes. Stir in the oats and cook for an extra minute, or until the mixture is smooth.

2. Serve the hot porridge with the sliced banana on top.

Nature delights in variety, and this cannot be any different when it comes to panning your diets. There are tons of delicious recipes out there that can make your day, and this manual contains just some of them. These recipes sustainable dietary option for you and you loved ones to enjoy!

☐

Chapter Six: Meal Plan

Since you have gotten to know almost everything about the Sirtfood diet, it is essential to introduce you to the meal plan. This is to bring you up to speed to understand how to achieve the most critical diet benefits.

As far as anyone knows, the Sirtfood diet includes nourishments that are generally plants containing an abundant quantity of a specific compound, known as sirtuins. Sirtuins activate genes that are responsible for burning fat. The eating regimen is broken down into two stages that are repeated consistently.

The primary stage includes living on only 1000 calories for three days and afterward on slightly more 1500 calories for four days. It also incorporates loads of consumption of green juices. The subsequent stage goes on for two weeks and includes three principle meals with loads of green juices.

From that point forward, you can keep an eating routine that contains Sirtfoods by including as much as possible Sirtfoods, not forgetting other ingredients.

The Seven-day Sirtfood Meal Plan

This is a 7-day meal plan incorporating the Sirtfood staples, including the healthy green juice and delicious choc balls.

Sirtfood Green Juice: This super-healthy juice that is to be taken three times daily in the first stage is made from kale (75g), rocket (30g), flat-leaf parsley (5g), celery (150g), a half medium apple, 1/2 lemon juice, 1/2 teaspoon of matcha green tea and lovage leaves (5g) which is optional.

Take note; however, that matcha is to be used in the initial two blends of the day since the caffeine content is similar to that of an ordinary teacup. In case you're not accustomed to it, it might keep you alert whenever you consume it later.

Sirtfood Bites: These are stuffed antioxidants, and they are made from blending walnuts (120g), dark chocolate (30g), pitted Medjool dates (250g), one tablespoon cocoa powder, one tablespoon ground turmeric, one tablespoon olive oil, and one tablespoon of vanilla concentrate or scraped seeds of a vanilla case.

Day 1
On the first day, you will take the Sirtfood green juice three times, the Sirtfood bites twice, and a Sirtfood meal. You may, however, substitute the Sirtfood bite for dark chocolate (15-20g).
Stir-fried Asian king prawn: Making this meal requires frying shelled king prawns (150g) in olive oil (2 tablespoons) with two tablespoon soy or tamari sauce, one finely chopped clove garlic, one finely chopped bird-eye chili, one finely chopped ginger, sliced red onions (20g), trimmed and sliced celery (40g), chopped green beans (75g), soba (75g) and celery leaves or lovage (5g).

Day 2
The second day also involves taking the Sirtfood green juice three times, the Sirtfood bites twice, and a Sirtfood meal.
Turkey escalope: Turkey escalope is prepared using ingredients such as roughly chopped cauliflower (150g), one finely chopped clove garlic, finely chopped red onion (40g), one finely chopped bird-eye chili, one tablespoon finely chopped fresh ginger, two tablespoons extra olive oil, two tablespoon ground turmeric, finely chopped sun-dried tomatoes (30g), parsley (10g), turkey escalope (150g), one tablespoon dried sage, 1/2 lemon juice and a tablespoon of capers.

Day 3
The third day involves the same routine as the first and second with Sirtfood green juice three times,

Sweet-smelling chicken: The turmeric contained in this meal serves the purpose of anti-inflammatory. The salsa is prepared from 1 enormous tomato, one finely cleaved bird-eye stew, one tablespoon of finely hacked escapades, finely slashed parsley (5g) 1/2 lemon juice. The chicken, on the other hand, is made from the boneless and skinned chicken breast (120g), two tablespoon ground turmeric, 1/2 lemon juice, one tablespoon additional olive oil, hacked kale (50g), cut red onion (20g), one tablespoon finely hacked new ginger and buckwheat (50g).

Day 4
On the fourth day, the Sirtfood green juice is reduced to twice with the Sirtfood bites and Sirtfood meal twice and once.
Sirt Muesli: This is an effortless meal, plus it offers a delicious beginning for the fourth day. The ingredients needed for this include buckwheat flakes (20g), buckwheat puffs (10g), coconut pieces (15g), pitted and cleaved Medjool dates (40g), chopped walnuts (15g), cocoa nibs (10g), hulled and cleaved strawberries (100g) and plain Greek yogurt (100g).
Sautéed Salmon Salad: Parsley (10g), 1/2 lemon juice, one tablespoon capers, and one tablespoon additional virgin olive oil are required for making the dressing. As for the salad, 1/2 peeled and diced avocado, split cherry tomatoes (100g), thinly cut red onion (20g), rocket (50g), celery leaves (5g), skinless salmon filet (150g), two tablespoons brown sugar, and split chicory (70g).

Day 5
The fifth day features Sirtfood green juice and Sirtfood meals twice each.
Strawberry tabbouleh: This is a dish that is super healthy as well as filling. The ingredients required for its preparation include buckwheat (50g), one tablespoon ground turmeric, avocado (80g), tomato (65g), red onion (20g), pitted Medjool dates (25g), one tablespoon escapades, parsley (30g), hulled strawberries (100g), one tablespoon additional olive oil, 1/2 lemon juice and rocket (30g).

Miso-marinated wild cod: This is a delicious cod dish and is capable of taking your mind off the feeling of being on a tight eating routine. The preparation requires ingredients such as miso (20g), one tablespoon mirin, one tablespoon additional olive oil, skinless cod filet (200g), cut red onion (20g), sliced celery (40g), one finely chopped clove garlic, one finely cut bird-eye chili, one tablespoon finely chopped ginger, green beans (60g), roughly chopped kale (50g), buckwheat (30g), one tablespoon ground turmeric, one tablespoon sesame seeds, roughly chopped parsley (5g) and one tablespoon soy or tamari sauce.

Day 6

Like the firth day, the sixth feature Sirtfood green juice and Sirtfood meals twice each.

Sirt salad: Sirt salad is prepared by mixing the ingredients. The ingredients are rocket (50g), chicory leaves (50g), smoked salmon cuts (100g), peeled and cut avocado (80g), cut celery (40g), cut red onion (20g), chopped walnut (15g), one tablespoon capers, one huge hollowed and cleaved Medjool date, one tablespoon additional olive oil, 1/2 lemon juice, chopped parsley (10g) and chopped celery or lovage leaves (10g).

Chargrilled meat: Peeled and cut potatoes (100g), one tablespoon additional olive oil, finely chopped parsley (5g), sliced red onion (50g), chopped kale (50g), one finely chopped clove garlic,

3.5cm-thick meat filet (120-150g), red wine (40ml), meat stock (150ml), one tablespoon tomato purée, and one tablespoon cornflour in one tablespoon water

Day 7

On the last day of the first stage, green juice is consumed twice and Sirtfood meals, which are consumed two times as well.

Sirtfood omelet: streaky bacon (50g), medium eggs (3), thinly cut red chicory (35g), finely chopped parsley (5g), and one tablespoon additional olive oil.

Chicken Breast (Baked): to prepare the pesto, you need parsley, walnuts, and Parmesan (15g each with one tablespoon additional olive oil and 1/2 lemon juice. To prepare the chicken, you would need skinless chicken (150g), finely cut red onions (20g), one tablespoon red wine vinegar, rocket (35g), split cherry tomatoes (100g), and one tablespoon balsamic vinegar.

The second stage goes on for about fourteen days. During this stage, you should keep on and shedding more weight consistently and get more fit. There isn't a particular limit to calories in this stage. Instead, you are to take a green juice per day and consume three meals brimming with Sirtfoods each day.

These two stages may be repeated as frequently as wanted for additional weight reduction. Be that as it may, you are urged to keep consuming Sirtfoods in your eating regimen after finishing these stages by including Sirtfoods in your meals consistently. There are also assortments of Sirtfoods, which you may incorporate into your eating regimen as snacks or plans you use already. Furthermore, you are urged to keep drinking the green squeeze each day. Along these lines, the diet turns out to be, to a greater extent, a change of your way of life change instead of a diet that you just consume one-time.

A Sirtfood Meal Plan

In light of these standards, this is what you could incorporate into your menu during the second stage in addition to the green squeezes.

Breakfast: For breakfast, you may take kale omelet, yogurt, and blueberries with muesli; or a fruit smoothie made from soy milk and rolled oats.

Lunch and Supper: For lunch or dinner, excellent options include spicy tofu that is packed with vegetables, stir-fried alongside bird-eye chili; rocket salad of mixed greens and fish, plus cucumbers and tomatoes served with olive oil on top of it; chicken and stir-fried soba noodles, buckwheat salad with grilled fish; wholegrain bread with tofu burgers and a plate of mixed greens, brown rice served with spicy chicken; or kale salad served alongside edamame beans with red onion served with olive oil.

Snacks and Bites: For snacks and bites, dark chocolate, coffee, celery, fresh fruits (especially apples, oranges and strawberries), and walnuts are great choices to choose from.

AT WHAT COSTS?
You truly need to design and approach the prescribed ingredients to follow this eating regimen appropriately. You'll likewise need to put resources into getting a conventional juicer, which may cost you at least $100. Strawberries and kale may be somewhat challenging to get at certain seasons. It's additionally hard to stick to when voyaging, at get-togethers, and taking care of a family that has small children.

The Sirtfood eating routine itself removes various nutritional categories and is constraining. Dairy nourishments, which give different essential supplements, including a few that most people need, aren't part of the arrangement. Also, matcha rich in polyphenol frequently contains lead as part of the tea leaves, which is possibly risky to your wellbeing, particularly when taken consistently. It also has a harsh flavor, just as 85% of dark chocolate, likewise suggested.

WHY THERE ARE NO SIRT SUPPLEMENTS
This is an inquiry that pops up consistently. Suppose sirtuins indeed are game-changers like we've been made to believe. Why are pharmaceutical companies and producers of supplements not making efforts to produce them and make them available in the form of pills?

This is because the component by which they sirtuins work despite everything isn't completely comprehended, implying that supplements will not be appropriately consumed like the natural form by the human body.

It is a better idea to devour a broad scope of these supplements as regular wholefoods, where they exist together near the many other normal bioactive substances that act cooperatively to help our wellbeing.

You can stick to this arrangement for as long as about fourteen days, after which you are free to alter the diet to go with your way of life. Set guidelines do not exist; attempt to incorporate as many Sirtfoods as could be allowed in your eating routine, which should cause you to feel more healthy, increasingly enthusiastic, improve the state of your skin, and making you slenderer.

Chapter Seven: How to improve the energy-boosting effect

From the previous chapters in this book, you have been exposed to the underlying idea, process, and food types involved in the Sirt Food diet. The remarkable health merits and the numerous benefits that your body stands the chance of getting have also been explained. However, in this chapter, we will discuss the strategies that can be used to improve the diet's energy-boosting effect.

As you have learned, the constituents and foods used in the diet are not outstanding calorific foods. The phase involved in following the diet also specifies the number of calories taken during each step. This should not be mistaken to mean that the diet restricts or deprives the body of adequate calorie supply. The total calorie intake for the first two days of the Sirt food diet amounts to 2500 calories. Therefore, the diet doesn't deprive you of energy but instead increases it. This chapter will focus on the strategies and methods that can be used to sustain the increase in life given by this diet and improve it during and after the Sirt food diet.

These strategies have nutritional and scientific backing. Hence you can be sure of a robust result if the steps are followed adequately.

1.   Do not stop eating highly nutritious foods.

The Sirt food diet is stacked with foods that increase the energy level and boost the calories consumed. This way, the body is not only provided with enough energy-giving food. It is also equipped with the required nutrients that allow the body to make fair use of these calories. An excellent way of maintaining the energy boost from the Sirt food diet is to keep taking these foods after the diet. While you don't have to continue eating Sirt foods, you should continue taking foods stacked with numerous nutrients, especially vitamins and minerals.

The importance of these two classes of food in the provision and maintenance of energy in the body has not been adequately discussed in recent times. The presence of vitamins and minerals in the body aids the optimum conversion of carbohydrate and other energy-giving foods to glucose, which is the body's primary energy source. Apart from helping the conversion process, it also allows for the body's ideal energy utilization. Hence, the energy boost derived from the Sirtfood can be sustained and improved by supplying the body with abundant nutrients, especially vitamins and minerals.

Foods that can supply these nutrients without affecting the calorie supply include grains, fruits, plants, and animal proteins and vegetables.

2 Ensure that you consume a lot of antioxidants

As a result of our daily activities and the types of food we consume, some chemicals are produced in the body. These chemicals are dangerous to our wellbeing as they induce stress and fatigue in the body, causing a large deletion of the body's energy—the best way of dealing with these energy-sapping chemicals through antioxidants.

Antioxidants are biochemical that eliminates these dangerous chemicals discussed above. However, these antioxidants are not produced in the body. Instead, they are supplied to the body through food, fruits, and some drugs. All of these sources of antioxidants provide the biochemical in different quantities and amounts.

The antioxidants naturally get from foods in massive quantities compared to those derived from processed foods or pills. If a comparative ratio is taken between the number of antioxidants called for foods and those gotten from drugs, you will find that it at a rate of 1000 to 1. Therefore, to increase the energy-boosting effect of the Sirt food diet, consume foods rich in antioxidants. Foods that are plant derivatives, vegetables, and fruits are excellent sources of antioxidants.

3 Avoid dieting or an unhealthy meal schedule.

You have just finished a Sirt food diet that has provided you with an impressive amount of energy. Starting another diet that will deplete this massive energy you have derived from the Sirt food diet should be avoided. This should not be misunderstood to mean that you cannot start another diet after the Sirt food diet. However, what is advised is that an in-depth study of the new diet should be done. This ensures that the modern diet doesn't involve foods or practices that will reduce the body's intake of necessary calories or nutrients.

Hence, to improve the energy-boosting effect that you are gaining from the Sirt food diet, you have to make sure that the daily calorific target as per the diet is met consistently. In both phases of the diet, you need to consume a stipulated amount of calories daily. These daily targets must be met.

Furthermore, after the completion of the Sirt food diet, ensure that sufficient amounts of energy-giving food are consumed. This is to ensure that the quantity of energy needed for your daily activities is provided.

4. Do not skip breakfast.

This strategy looks a lot like the previous one, but in essence, it is not. Most people are making it a habit to miss the first meal of the day due to a busy schedule or other reasons. While it is true that skipping breakfast might help you save time, it is also an unhealthy habit in the long run, especially for those who work for several hours and those who do strenuous jobs.

Breakfast is one of, if not the most important meal of the day. This is so because it provides the body with the required energy to start the day. Nutritionists and dieticians have often advised that an adequate quantity of carbohydrates should be present in your breakfast. The rationale behind this advice is that a fair amount of carbohydrates will produce a sufficient amount of energy for the human body to carry out various activities before noon.

By skipping this critical meal, the body is deprived of a necessary dose of energy that it requires. This depletes the energy reserve of the body and causes a sensation of lethargy. For people who are just ending the Sirt food diet, where an adequate amount of energy has been provided for the body, skipping breakfast feels like a relapse. This is because all the energy-boosting effect that the diet has added to the body is lost. One way to improve the Sirt food diet's energy-boosting effect is to ensure that you take your breakfast regularly.

5 Hydration
Water is an integral part of human life. This importance is also extended to human health and nutrition. The human body requires a considerable amount of water to enable it to work in an optimum condition. Different activities and processes in the body require lots of water. Hence, the importance of hydration cannot be overemphasized in the body.
About the improvement of energy in the body, hydration also plays an essential role. To avoid any form of misconception, drinking water and hydrating the body doesn't provide the body with energy, except energy drinks. However, hydrating the body enables the bodywork optimally, which means that processes like metabolism are carried out efficiently. When metabolism is carried out efficiently, the body is provided with an adequate amount of energy.
Therefore, during and after the Sirt food diet, ensure that your body is sufficiently hydrated to keep up the diet's energy level.
6 Avoid Alcohol
Among other things, alcohol is a powerful source of energy depletion in the body. This is because alcohol acts in two ways in the body. The first action is as a depressant. Alcohol lowers the body processes, including metabolism. This, in turn, results in a reduction in the production of energy for body activities.

Alcohol also acts as a stimulant in the body. In this way, it causes a hyper sensation or feeling in the body, thereby raising the rate of somebody's processes. Although this high rate of body processes increases the metabolism rate, which may result in a boost in energy, it also disturbs the sleeping schedule. A disrupted sleeping cycle will translate into a tired and lethargic body, reducing power in the body.

Therefore, to maintain and improve the energy-boosting effect of the Sirt food diet, it is advised that the consumption of alcohol should be reduced to the barest minimum. If you are still on the Sirt food diet, you can replace alcohol drinks with red wine, which has a controlled amount of alcohol and possesses some antioxidants.

7 Watch your caffeine intake.

Just like alcohol, caffeine also has a stimulating effect on the body. This way, there is an upsurge of energy after the consumption of caffeinated drinks. However, this energizing effect is short-term as it wears off after some time. The aftermath of this non-lasting energizer is fatigue and hunger. As a result, you tend to overeat and consume an unhealthy amount of calories or sugar to cater to the energy loss and lethargic sensation. And that is not a very good thing, especially if you are still undertaking the Sirt food diet.

Caffeine can be used seldom and with caution to avoid addiction or overdependence. This controlled use of caffeine is one way by which the energy-boosting effect of the Sirt food diet can be improved.

Another option that should be considered, especially when addiction or reliance on caffeine is noticed, is green tea. Green tea is an excellent source of theanine, a useful chemical that helps calm the body and retain focus. Green tea is also a perfect option for those still undergoing the Sirt food diet and those just ending the diet. This is because it is a healthy source of antioxidants, whose importance has been explained earlier.

8 Smart snacks

It has been said that the body needs a constant source of energy throughout the day to avoid lethargy and fatigue from setting in. The healthiest source of this energy is real food throughout the day. However, the reality is that most people cannot afford to eat real food when they need their energy boost due to work and other related factors. This brings the idea of fast foods and snacks. But ironically, most of the snacks available in most cases are not healthy sources of energy either. They either contain too much fat or too much sugar or leave the body with more health and energy complications. They don't provide the needed amount of energy except for a short-lived supply of strength, which will later leave the body tired. This is where smart snacks come into play.

Smart snacks are snacks made from fruits, nuts, vegetables, and other nutritious foods. The idea behind the intelligent snack innovation is to combine appropriate amounts of fats, protein, and other nutrients that can be found in the fruits and foods mentioned above. By combining these foods and fruits in a snack, energy is not only healthily provided for the body, but the release of this energy is controlled to maximize its power without suffering a depletion.

Therefore, another strategy for ensuring that the energy-boosting effects of the Sirtfood are sustained and improved upon even after the diet is snack smartly. The consumption of smart snacks holds many health benefits for the body, even outside improvement of the Sirt food diet's energy-boosting effect.

These eight methods that are explained in these chapters are tested and trusted to maintain your energy level even without the Sirt food diet. However, with the Sirt food diet, your body has acquired lots of energy from its nutritional content. It is only logical to sustain these energy levels and improve on it to ensure that the effect of the Sirt food diet lasts long.

□

Chapter Eight: Guide on how to start and maintain the Sirtfood diet

Now that you have learned about almost everything there is to learn about the Sirtfood diet, let's get you started. Starting a diet requires some forms of preparation to ensure that the time and resources invested in the diet are not wasted. This chapter will give out essential tips that will help you start the Sirtfood diet on a good note and help you maintain the diet.

To begin with, let's give tips that will help you kick off the Sirtfood diet in an appropriate manner.

Consult a health/medical practitioner

Before starting the Sirtfood diet, you must see your doctor or dietician first. People have different health and underlying medical conditions. These conditions affect the amount, types, and quality of nutrients in the body. And since the bulk of our nutrients are gotten from the food we eat, it is only necessary that we ensure that we do not miss or reduce the number of nutrients we ingest.

Checking in with your medical practitioner, especially one you are familiar with over a long period and has your medical history, ensures that all the necessary considerations are taken care of before you start the Sirtfood diet. Meeting with the doctor will help you know the foods that you should and should not avoid at a particular time due to your health conditions. The dietician can help analyze the foods involved in the diet and advise if it is safe for you to start with the diet or not. If there is a need to change certain foods in the diet, the dietician can help you provide appropriate alternatives without undermining the diet's effectiveness.

Therefore, one of the crucial steps that you should take is meeting with health professionals for guidance and adequate information about the Sirtfood diet before you start.

Draw up your targets

You are starting the Sirtfood diet for specific reasons. It could be to lose unhealthy fat and weight healthily or obtain a rejuvenated energy boost for your daily activities. It could be both of these benefits or even more. You must draw out your goals and target before starting the Sirtfood diet. Drawing out your Sirtfood diet goals has many benefits, especially for the auspicious beginning and maintenance of the diet.

By setting your diet goals, you have a clear picture of what you intend to achieve at the end of the Sirtfood diet. It gives you a clear image of what you want to look like, how you want to feel, and the benefits you wish to amass by the end of the diet. This clear picture of the future you at the end of the Sirtfood diet is a fantastic inspiration source. This motivation is a necessary tool for starting the diet. It keeps you going and motivates you when you feel like stopping or relapsing.

Apart from motivating you and helping you with confidence when you feel like stopping, drawing out your diet goals has other advantages. It helps you define pathways and processes during the diet. These defined processes make it easy to start and stick to the Sirtfood diet.

Make realistic goals

This step is more like a sequel to the last step. There is another crucial step after understanding the importance of drawing up your diet goals and the benefits you wish to derive from the diet after completion. This involves making realistic goals. It is not sufficient to set dreams and visions; it is also essential to ask if those goals are reasonably attainable.

By making realistic and attainable goals, you are doing yourself a lot of good regarding the success of the diet. Firstly, it helps with the morale-boosting necessary for the inception of the diet. Knowing fully well that the goals you set are realistically attainable, the energy and motivation to start the diet are peaks. The mind will look forward to the target, thus helping the bodywork tirelessly towards it.

Setting realistic goals before starting the Sirtfood diet helps you stick to the diet. This point can better be explained using a scenario where an unrealistic goal has been set. After a long sticking to the diet without achieving these goals (which is very likely since the goals are unrealistic), the mind becomes discouraged, and the body feels weary. Such a person sees no need to continue sticking to the diet since he/she erroneously believes that the diet couldn't help achieve the desired goals. Setting realistic diet goals before starting the Sirtfood diet is as essential as every other tip given before.

Change your pantry/store.

You are about to take one of the crucial steps in your life, deciding to start the Sirtfood diet. Hence you need the right and necessary resources. It is not enough to prepare yourself mentally and psychologically. Physical preparation is also essential. And by physical practice, I am referring to the food and utensils you will need to start and complete the Sirtfood diet successfully. So clearing out your pantry and replenishing it with needed food items and fruits is an important step.

Unhealthy foods or foods that do not align with the Sirtfood diet content should be taken out of the house. This helps you focus on the diet and, in the long run, enables you to maintain the diet by avoiding relapses. If you are staying with family or relatives who are not starting the Sirtfood diet, communicate with them about your diet plans and why you need to avoid them. This will help them to plan how to keep these unhealthy foods out of your sight. Remember, out of sight is out of mind.

After clearing the pantry, replacing it with the needed food items is the next step. You already know the foods that are required for the Sirtfood diet. Stock up your food storage with these foods, fruits, and beverages as the case may be. There may also be a need to add new kitchen utensils to your kitchen. Get these utensils so that the preparation of the foods in the Sirtfood diet is made easy.

Talk to your family and friends.

Although this point was briefly mentioned in the previous step, there is a need to elaborate on it. If you are staying with your family or friends, there is a need to talk to them about your plans to start the Sirtfood diet. Let them know your reasons and motivations for starting the diet. And ultimately, let them know how they can support you during and after the inception of the diet.

Support from family and friends is very crucial to the success of the Sirtfood diet. Apart from helping you avoid unhealthy foods, they can remind you of your goals and target and keep you motivated through the diet course. Also, telling your friends and family about the Sirtfood diet and what you intend to gain at the end may inspire some of them to join you. This is a massive boost for your morale during the diet as you and these friends can help each other stay on track and avoid relapses.

Get a dieting partner.

This tip is taken from the last point and will be discussed briefly. Getting a dieting partner helps with morale boost at the beginning of the diet. You can share your plans, body reactions, and difficulties experienced during the diet. You can also encourage each other during the Sirtfood diet.

These tips are essential tips that will help your kickstart your Sirtfood diet successfully. The information should be followed as much as possible.

Maintaining the Sirtfood Diet

After the successful beginning of the Sirtfood diet, there is more work to do. There is a need to ensure that the morale and momentum you had at the beginning of the diet are maintained to complete the diet. The tips given in this regard have been tested and confirmed to help people manage the motivation and morale for completing the Sirtfood diet.

Check-in with your set goals.

You have understood the importance of setting goals at the inception of the Sirtfood diet. We have discussed that these goals need to attainable and realistic to allow for adherence to it. However, these realistic goals that you have set need to be checked continuously during the diet. Continually checking in with your set goals reminds you of the reason for starting the diet in the first place. It brings up the image of the future you had in mind at the beginning of the Sirtfood diet. By checking your set target during the diet course, the primary source of motivation and inspiration for the diet is revived, thus giving you enough will continue with the Sirtfood diet no matter the difficulties encountered.

Apart from reviving the motivation for continuing the Sirtfood diet, reviewing your goals allows you to track your progress concerning the diet. Remember that while drawing up your plans, the processes and pathways are also defined. These defined pathways are used to monitor your progress with the Sirtfood diet.

Understand that it acceptable to make mistakes

One of the banes of most dieters is cheating or eating off-plan. This occurs when they eat foods that are not in tandem with the dictates of their diet. In the Sirtfood diet, it is possible to eat off-plan too. There are days you may overeat or eat wrongly due to forgetfulness, and some days you may just give in to your cravings. If and when any of these occasions, do not be too hard on yourself and do not lose hope. You need to remember that you are only human, and it is acceptable to make mistakes. Most importantly, you must remember that the most vital and helpful step you can take after eating out of the diet is to pick up yourself and learn from your mistakes.

You need to understand the reason for the relapse. Was it due to cravings or forgetfulness? What exactly went wrong? Getting answers to these questions will help you map out the steps that you must take to avoid such relapse next time. For instance, if the mistake was due to forgetfulness, you can set up periodic reminders to always keep you in check at all times.

On the other hand, if the mistake was born out of cravings, you may need to talk to your dietician. The dietician will help you find out if the food items you are craving can hurt the Sirtfood diet plans. This will help provide options and solutions to overcome this mistake.

In summary, after making a mistake with the diet plan, the next course of action should be how to overcome the error and prevent future occurrences.

Combine exercises with the Sirtfood Diet

Exercises are very beneficial to human health. Combining it with a healthy diet like the Sirtfood diet increases the health benefits that can be derived. However, exercising regularly during the diet has immense health benefits and helps you stay focused on a diet. You may wonder how that works.

By combining exercise with the Sirtfood diet, there is a considerable likelihood of quickly and easily achieving your set goals. For people going into the Sirtfood diet to achieve healthy weight loss, exercising is a great plus that quickly achieves this goal. Also, exercises help you accomplish this accessible for people going into the diet for the energy-boosting effect.

When your set goals are achieved easily during the Sirtfood diet, the zeal to remain focused and maintain the diet is renewed. The possibility of getting discouraged during the dieting process is reduced as you can see the diet's achievements.

Smart Snacking

While on a diet such as the Sirtfood diet, there is a restriction on what to eat and drink. Hence, in situations where you need to be away from home for an extended period, you need to ensure that you have a reliable source of Sirtfoods to eat when the need arises. Because it is not very comfortable to pack food items with you wherever you go, snacks remain the best and most suitable option.

Snacks and fast food are handy in serving as an alternative to real foods when the need arises. However, not all snacks can be used in place of Sirtfoods. This is the origination of the concept of smart snacks. The idea of intelligent snacks was discussed in detail in the previous chapter.

Smart snacks are healthy and appropriate alternatives that can be used in place of Sirtfoods, especially when you are away from home or cannot access your Sirtfood items. Snacking is another way of maintaining the Sirtfood diet. By having smart snacks on you whenever you are far from home, you have the opportunity to feed your body with needed nutrients through the smart snack without eating unhealthy food or out of the Sirtfood diet.

Make the best out of your restaurant time.

Sometimes, it is impossible to have access to smart snacks, as advised in the previous tip. It may be due to forgetfulness on your part, or you cannot afford to get some because of time or space. In most cases, the only option you are left with at this point is to eat out or starve until you get home. Of course, starving yourself is not an ideal option as it undermines your strength to carry out your work and other activities effectively.

The viable choice here is to eat at a restaurant. As discouraging as it may sound to your Sirtfood diet plan, you can still attempt to make the best out of it. Make inquiries about the availability of some Sirtfoods in the restaurant. While some particular foods are peculiar to the Sirtfood diet, some general food items are also sirtuin-friendly. Try to get these foods if you can.

However, if these foods are not available, opt-in for nutritious or healthy foods; although these foods are not Sirtfoods, they are filled with essential nutrients that will do your body a whole lot of good. Some of these foods are also discussed in detail in the previous chapter. If these foods and fruits are available at your eat-out spot or restaurant, they are safe for you to eat.

If the restaurants do not have these types of food in stock, you can eat whatever pleases you on the menu. This is the next best option other than starving yourself. However, you must bear in mind that you need to balance this episode of eating out with sufficient Sirtfoods so that your goals are not affected.

Mind what you eat

There is a practice called mindful eating. It involves people paying detailed and intricate attention to what they eat and its effect on their bodies. To some school of thought, mindful eating is a diet with some health benefits. While I will not precisely classify mindful eating as a diet type, there is no doubt that it has some advantages, health-wise. These benefits, among other things, will help you stay focused on your Sirtfood diet.

By practicing mindful eating, the body is put in a position to receive more nutrients and less unhealthy elements. This is because mindful eating requires researching thoroughly into the nutritional constituents of what we eat. By doing so, nutritious and beneficial foods are distinguished from unhealthy food. Since it is unlikely that anyone would knowingly consume unhealthy foods, more nutrients are fed into the body by eating healthy foods.

Feeding the body with enough nutrients helps maintain the Sirtfood diet. With abundant nutrient in the body, the benefits of the diet can easily be achieved and sustained. Therefore, if you wish to maintain the Sirtfood diet, you can practice mindful eating to help with the process.

Stick to the Sirtfood Diet Plan

This point sounds like a no-brainer, but it is crucial and requires reiteration. Sticking to the diet plan is one sure way of ensuring that both short term and long term goals of the diet are achieved.

Sticking to the diet plan from the inception of the Sirtfood diet is instrumental in attaining the short-term goals. These goals include drastic but healthy weight loss and improvement in the body's energy level, among other things. Apart from their inherent health benefits, the attainment of these goals is a significant boost to the morale of anyone undertaking the diet. Seeing that some of the goals set at the beginning of the diet have been achieved, remaining focused and maintaining the diet would be less stressful. Hence sticking to the diet plan is a vital step in ensuring that you retain the Sirtfood diet.

Furthermore, the success of all the tips previously given is dependent on your ability to stick with the diet plan. Without the determination to stick to the diet plan, all the other suggestions will be useless and ineffective.
These tips given below help you maintain the zeal and momentum for the Sirtfood diet. This way, the successful completion of the dieting process is ensured.

☐

Conclusion

The Sirtfood diet is the latest dietary innovation that the world is still talking about at the moment. Some celebrities' impressive weight loss has been linked to the diet makes the discussions more interesting and widespread. However, the idea and science behind the concept have been explained. The polyphenol action in the Sirtfood items regarding the production and activation of the sirtuins has been defined. It so has the effect of the calorific reduction in the diet.

It is important to note that despite the numerous benefits associated with the diet, medical practitioners have raised concerns about the effectiveness of the diet. The issues they raised related to the calorie intake restrictions and the number of Sirtfoods to be consumed in the diet. To this end, it is advised that you consult your doctor or dietician before adopting the diet. This will help you determine whether it is safe to start the diet and whether there is a need to make some exceptions to the Sirtfood diet requirements as demanded by your health condition.

Conclusively, the Sirtfood diet is a fantastic diet with many advantages to the health of the adopters. From healthily losing weight to increasing the body's energy reserve, there are many benefits that you stand to gain when you stick to the Sirtfood diet.

About the Author

Maria Baker is an experienced nutritionist originally from the United Kingdom. In his career spanning over two decades, the published author has helped coach thousands across the globe to understand their issues about wellness and researching the best ways to lead healthy with her diet plans including the Sirtfood Diet.

She works closely with healthcare organizations in devising diet plans. Many of her patients have achieved amazing results as fat loss, increased lean mass, and physical health with her diet plans.

She wrote a Sirtfood Diet book to help as many people as possible with her unique recipes. In her book you will learn all you need to know about this diet to get the best results from it.